Infection Protection: Pandemic

Ronald Klatz, M.D., D.O.
President, American Academy of Anti-Aging Medicine (A4M)

and

Robert Goldman, M.D., Ph.D., D.O., FAASP
Chairman, American Academy of Anti-Aging Medicine (A4M)
Chairman, International Medical Commission

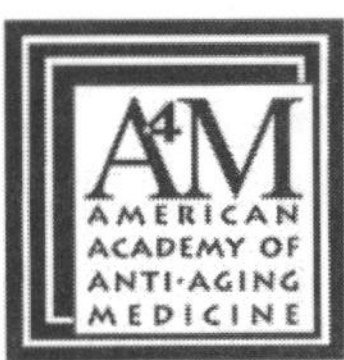

American Academy of Anti-Aging Medicine (A4M)
www.worldhealth.net

IMPORTANT: PLEASE READ

The content presented in *Infection Protection: Pandemic* is for educational purposes only and is not intended to prevent, diagnose, treat or cure disease or illness. While potentially therapeutic pharmaceuticals, nutraceuticals (dietary supplementation) and interventive therapies are mentioned in the course of this book, you are urged to seek the advice of a qualified medical professional to determine the appropriateness for your particular medical condition.

Dosing of nutraeuticals can be highly variable. Proper dosing is based on parameters including sex, age, and whether the patient is well or ill (and, if ill, whether it is a chronic or acute situation). Additionally, efficiency of absorption of a particular type of product and the quality of its individual ingredients are two major considerations for choosing appropriate specific agents for an individual's medical situation. Anyone on prescription medication should first consult their physician prior to starting any new therapy, including nutraceuticals. Furthermore, anyone with malignancy should consult their physician or oncologist prior to beginning, or continuing, any hormone therapy program.

Please be mindful that just because a product is natural doesn't mean it's safe for everyone. A small portion of the general population may react adversely to components in nutraceuticals (especially botanical products). Make your physician aware of any and all interventions you use regularly, and seek medical consultation before starting any others.

Neither the publisher nor the authors advocate the use of any particular healthcare protocol or therapeutic agent, but believe this information in this book should be available to the public. The publisher and authors are not responsible for any adverse effects resulting from use of any of the suggestions, preparations, or procedures discussed in this book. **Always consult your physician prior to beginning any new healthcare regimen, whether it be nutritional, fitness, medication, hormonal, herbal, or otherwise. Do not change your existing regimen without discussing with your physician first.**

For those individuals interested in learning more about the suggestions, preparations, or procedures mentioned in this book, the publisher and authors urges that you consult a knowledgeable physician or health practitioner, preferably one who has been Board Certified in Anti-Aging Medicine. You may find one by utilizing the Online Physician/Practitioner Locator at the educational website of the American Academy of Anti-Aging Medicine (A4M), www.worldhealth.net, or you may call the A4M's international headquarters in Chicago, IL USA at (773) 528-4333.

Chief Researcher and Editor: Catherine Cebula
Assistant Researcher: Lindsay Steel
Cover Design: Robert Buzek Designs

Printed in the United States of America.

Contents

Online updates at: www.worldhealth.net/pandemic

Pandemic: Not a question of *"if,"* but *"when"* ...
English Clergyman Thomas Fuller (1608-1661) remarked: "In fair weather prepare for foul." A prudent individual will prepare for disaster before it is on the doorstep.

Log on to **www.worldhealth.net/pandemic** every week to read the latest tips for protecting yourself and your loved ones from the wrath of an impending infectious disease outbreak.

Preface

A pandemic is a global disease outbreak. An influenza pandemic occurs when a new influenza A virus emerges for which there is little or no immunity in the human population, begins to cause serious illness, and then spreads easily person-to-person worldwide. Scientists are concerned that the bird flu virus — H5N1 — one day could be able to infect humans and spread easily from one person to another, because we have no existing immunity to the disease. If H5N1 virus were to gain the capacity to spread easily from person to person, an influenza pandemic — the worldwide outbreak of disease — could begin.

Experts vary widely on projections of the numbers of people who would become ill and the numbers who would die. Historically, we can refer to the 1918-1919 influenza pandemic, which is often referred to as "America's forgotten pandemic," as a frame of reference. Historians estimate that, at one point, over half of the 1.6 billion people in the world in 1918 were infected with the Spanish Flu. Millions of young, healthy adults fell ill to the disease and died from the suffocation it caused. Experts now estimate that approximately 80 to 100 million people perished worldwide, and at least 500,000 Americans died. Not only reducing the global population by one-sixteenth, the 1918 flu pandemic caused brain damage in many of its survivors. The 1918 flu pandemic caused the largest one-year decline in the average lifespan in the United States in modern history, slashing it by a full twelve years.

The worst-case scenario:

- Worldwide, the United Nations estimates that from **5 to 150 million** people may die should an H5N1 pandemic occur. The World Health Organization projects from **2 million to 7.4 million** deaths, which it concedes is a "relatively conservative estimate" for purposes of providing a plausible planning target. The World Bank cites sources suggesting that a more virulent form (similar to the 1918-1919 strain) of pandemic flu may kill as many as **180–260 million** in a worst-case scenario.

- In preparing its Implementation Plan for the National Strategy for Pandemic Influenza, the U.S. federal government assumes that 30% of the population — 100 million — would be infected, and that as many as **1.9 million** would die — greater than the total deaths caused in a single year by heart disease, cancers, strokes, chronic pulmonary disease, AIDS, and Alzheimer's Disease combined. One disease model projects that if the U.S. population (standing at 295 million at the time of the projection) is exposed to the H5N1 flu strain, 33% would be infected (97.3 million) with a resulting death rate of 0.58% (**5.6 million** deaths) — more than twice the number of deaths from all the ten leading causes of death combined. So far, however, H5N1 has been 57% lethal in humans, meaning that in the very-worst case, possibly **upwards of 50 million** Americans may die.

The best-case scenario: An H5N1 pandemic strikes but is no more lethal than seasonal influenza. Be mindful, however, that even this scenario has a sizeable death toll — 200,000 to 1.5 million deaths worldwide and 36,000 in the U.S. alone.

Death rates from pandemic are largely determined by four factors: the number of people who become infected, the virulence of the virus, the underlying characteristics and vulnerability of affected populations, and the effectiveness of preventive measures. Accurate predictions of mortality cannot be made before the pandemic virus emerges and begins to spread. Of course, all estimates of the number of deaths are purely speculative. But it is important to know the scenario endpoints so you can prepare and protect yourself appropriately.

Infectious disease experts agree that it's not "if" bird flu will enter the United States, but "when." The resulting H5N1 pandemic will cripple the US economy, halting most commerce for a period of 12 to 24 months and bankrupting the federal government and most American citizens. The pandemic will also cause grave panic among the nation's residents, as sources of food, medicine, and the necessities of daily living will ultimately become unavailable. Presently, there is little effective, unified worldwide or national leadership in the arena of discovering real prevention and/or treatment protocols for H5N1. Consequently, it is up to each of us as individuals, to mount our own personal preparedness and protection program. In *Infection Protection: Pandemic* we outline a set of Top Ten Preventive Strategies against a backdrop of information about bird flu and its current — and potentially fatal future — ramifications.

As physicians we also ask you to be mindful to the recent upward trend in deaths due to respiratory diseases. In the U.S., influenza and pneumonia are now the 7th leading cause of death (responsible for 2.7% of all deaths in the nation), and chronic lower respiratory diseases are now are the 4th leading cause of death (5.1% of all U.S. deaths). All totaled these diseases kill more than 190,000 Americans each year.

A direct threat to how long and well you live, respiratory diseases are largely avoidable and preventable. In writing *Infection Protection: Pandemic,* we seek to achieve three goals. First, our "best case" scenario is to aim to help you protect and strengthen your immune system so it is better able to ward off infectious pathogens of all kinds. Secondly, our "worst case" scenario is for this book to provide essential strategies for you — and your loved ones — to deploy in the event of a potential bird flu pandemic. Lastly, *Infection Protection: Pandemic* is designed to serve as a personal survival handbook for the certain to-come influenza, cold, and respiratory infectious disease epidemics that are an annual inevitable and unavoidable part of our everyday lives.

Enjoy this book in good health.
Ronald Klatz, M.D., D.O.
Robert Goldman, M.D., Ph.D., D.O., FAASP
Chicago, Illinois USA
June 2006

Chapter 1. Scenario Snapshot

Current Situation

Infection in humans by avian influenza — caused by the H5N1 virus, was first recognized in 1997 when this virus infected 18 people in Hong Kong, causing 6 deaths. Concern has increased in recent years as avian H5N1 infections have killed large numbers of poultry flocks and other birds in Asia, Europe, and Africa. Since 2003 and as of 6 June 2006, the World Health Organization (WHO) has tabulated a total of 225 human cases of H5N1 influenza affecting 10 nations. With 128 resulting deaths, H5N1 has a 57% death rate:

Country	2003		2004		2005		2006		Total	
	Cases	Deaths	Cases	Deaths	Cases	Deaths	Cases	Deaths	Cases	Deaths
Azerbaijan	0	0	0	0	0	0	8	5	8	5
Cambodia	0	0	0	0	4	4	2	2	6	6
China	0	0	0	0	8	5	10	7	18	12
Djibouti	0	0	0	0	0	0	1	0	1	0
Egypt	0	0	0	0	0	0	14	6	14	6
Indonesia	0	0	0	0	17	11	32	26	49	37
Iraq	0	0	0	0	0	0	2	2	2	2
Thailand	0	0	17	12	5	2	0	0	22	14
Turkey	0	0	0	0	0	0	12	4	12	4
Vietnam	3	3	29	20	61	19	0	0	93	42
Total	3	3	46	32	95	41	81	52	225	128

Source: "Cumulative Number of Confirmed Human Cases of Avian Influenza (H5N1) Reported to WHO," World Health Organization Epidemic and Pandemic Alert and Response, 6 June 2006, http://www.who.int/csr/disease/avian_influenza/country/cases_table_2006_06_06/en/index.html.

The main risks for human health from avian influenza are twofold:
1) The risk of direct infection when the virus passes from the infected bird to humans, sometimes resulting in severe disease;
2) The risk that the virus – if given enough opportunities – will change into a form that is highly infectious for humans and spreads easily from person to person.

Of the few avian influenza viruses that have crossed the species barrier to infect humans, H5N1 has caused the largest number of detected cases of severe disease and death in humans. <u>In the current outbreaks in Asia and Europe more than half of those infected with the virus have died. Most cases have occurred in previously healthy children and young adults.</u>

So far, the spread of H5N1 virus from person to person has been limited. Notable findings of epidemiologic investigations of human H5N1 cases in Vietnam during 2005 have suggested transmission of H5N1 viruses to at least two persons through consumption of uncooked duck blood. In 2004, in Thailand, there was evidence of probable human-to-human transmission between an ill child and her mother, who engaged in prolonged very close contact; transmission did not continue beyond one person. An extended family cluster of H5N1 infection was discovered in May 2006 in Indonesia. In this case, 8 members of the family contracted bird flu, resulting with 7 deaths. The World Health Organization (WHO) established that the initial case, a 37-year old woman, sold fruits at a market stand 45 feet (15 meters) from where live chickens were sold. She also kept a few chickens in her home, three of which died before she became ill. The family purchased chickens and pigs that were positive for H5 antibodies, from a nearby village. All confirmed cases in the family cluster spent their time together – mostly in one room, and experienced close and prolonged exposure to the initial patient during a severe phase of her illness. WHO considers this situation to reflect limited human-to-human transmission. WHO does not consider this Indonesian cluster to be a case of efficient (easily transmitted) and sustained human-to-human transmission that represents pandemic risk.

Nonetheless, because all influenza viruses have the ability to change, scientists are concerned that H5N1 virus one day could be able to infect humans and spread easily from one person to another. Because the virus does not commonly infect humans, there is little or no immune protection against them in the human population. If H5N1 were to gain the capacity to spread easily from person to person, an influenza pandemic (worldwide outbreak of disease) could begin.

Many scientists believe it is a matter of time until the next influenza pandemic occurs. However, the timing and severity of the next pandemic cannot be predicted. Although it is unpredictable when the next pandemic will occur and what strain may cause it, the continued and expanded spread of a highly pathogenic—and now endemic—avian H5N1 virus across eastern Asia and other countries represents a significant threat. No one can predict when a pandemic might occur. However, experts from around the world are watching the H5N1 situation in Asia and Europe very closely and are preparing for the possibility that the virus may begin to spread more easily and widely from person to person.

Migratory birds, the poultry trade, and human travel are among the possible mechanisms that experts believe could introduce pandemic flu into the United States.

The H5N1 virus has raised concerns about a potential human pandemic because:

1. The H5N1 virus is widespread in poultry in many countries in Asia and has spread to Europe and Africa;
2. The virus has been transmitted from birds to mammals and in some limited circumstances to humans;
3. Wild birds and domestic ducks have been infected without showing symptoms and become carriers of viral infection to other domestic poultry species;
4. A few cases of human-to-human transmission have been reported; and
5. Genetic studies confirm that H5N1 influenza viruses, like other influenza viruses, are continuing to evolve.

Although H5N1 probably poses the greatest current pandemic threat, other avian influenza A subtypes also have infected people in recent years. For example, in 1999, H9N2 infections were identified in Hong Kong; in 2002 and 2003, H7N7 infections occurred in the Netherlands and H7N3 infections occurred in Canada. These viruses also have the potential to give rise to the next pandemic.

Potential Pandemic

Pandemic flu is caused by a new influenza virus that people have not been exposed to before. It is likely to be more severe, affect more people, and cause more deaths than seasonal flu because people will not have immunity to the new virus. Symptoms of pandemic flu may be similar to the common flu, but frequently are more severe with complications more serious. Healthy adults may be at increased risk for serious complications. Pandemic flu differs from seasonal flu in several important ways:

Characteristic	Seasonal Flu	Pandemic Flu
Deaths	Average U.S. deaths approximately 36,000/year	Number of deaths could be quite high (for example, the U.S. 1918 death toll was approximately 500,000)
Symptoms	Symptoms: fever, cough, runny nose, muscle pain. Deaths often caused by complications, such as pneumonia.	Symptoms may be more severe and complications more frequent
		(continued)

Outbreak Frequency	Outbreaks follow predictable seasonal patterns; occurs annually, usually in winter, in temperate climates	Occurs rarely (three times in 20th century - most recently, in 1968)
Immunity	Usually some immunity built up from previous exposure	No previous exposure; little or no pre-existing immunity
Who's At Risk	Healthy adults usually not at risk for serious complications; the very young, the elderly and those with certain underlying health conditions at increased risk for serious complications	Healthy people may be at increased risk for serious complications
Health Systems Support	Health systems can usually meet public and patient needs	Health systems may be overwhelmed
Vaccine Availability	Vaccine developed based on known flu strains and available for annual flu season	Vaccine probably would not be available in the early stages of a pandemic
Anti-Virals Availability	Adequate supplies of antivirals are usually available	Effective antivirals may be in limited supply
Effect on Society	Generally causes modest impact on society (for example, some school closing, encouragement of people who are sick to stay home)	May cause major impact on society (for example, widespread restrictions on travel, closings of schools and businesses, cancellation of large public gatherings)
Effect on Economy	Manageable impact on domestic and world economy	Potential for severe impact on domestic and world economy

A Brief History of Contemporary Pandemic Events

A pandemic is a global disease outbreak. Pandemic influenza is virulent human flu that causes a global outbreak — a pandemic — of serious illness. Because there is little natural immunity, the disease can spread easily from person to person. A flu pandemic occurs when a new influenza virus emerges for which people have little or no immunity, and for which there is no vaccine. The disease spreads easily person-to-person, causes serious illness, and can sweep across the country and around the world in very short time. A pandemic may come and go in waves, each of which can last for six to eight weeks.

Currently, there is no pandemic flu. It is difficult to predict when the next influenza pandemic will occur or how severe it will be. Wherever and whenever a pandemic starts, everyone around the world is at risk. Countries might, through measures such as border closures and travel restrictions, delay arrival of the virus, but cannot stop it.

Historically, the 20th century saw 3 pandemics of influenza, each caused by a new strain of the influenza virus that spread wildly worldwide:

- 1918-1919 Most severe. Caused at least 500,000 U.S. deaths and 80 to 100 million deaths worldwide.
- 1957-1958 Moderately severe. Caused at least 70,000 U.S. deaths and 1 to 2 million deaths worldwide.
- 1968-1969 Least severe. Caused at least 34,000 U.S. deaths and 700,000 deaths worldwide.

The Potential H5N1 Pandemic

The virus that causes bird flu — H5N1 — has fulfilled three of four conditions that define a pandemic:

- ☑ 1. The H5N1 virus, pathogenic for humans, has established a global presence in a host population
- ☑ 2. The H5N1 virus is new in people
- ☑ 3. The virus has infected people, and they get seriously ill — H5N1 has a 50%+ mortality rate

H5N1 need only fulfill one more condition to become categorized as a pandemic:

4. The virus spreads easily from person to person

If H5N1 mutates into an easily transmissible virus before vaccine and anti-viral production and supplies are sufficient to treat a significant proportion of the worldwide population, no one will be immune from it.

Most experts think pandemic strains originate in birds or other animals. Dr. Ann Reid and Dr. Jeffery Taubenberger, of the Armed Forces Institute of Pathology recently wrote, "it is important to recognize that the mechanisms by which pandemic strains originate have not been explained yet." Furthermore, there is a persistent theory that influenza lies dormant in humans, not birds or swine, where it mutates into a killer strain. Some species have the misfortune to be about halfway between birds and humans. Pigs, for example, are susceptible to both avian and human strains of flu. What scientists fear is that a pig somewhere may be infected with both viruses at the same time. With proteins and RNA strands from both viruses floating around inside the cell, new viruses might assemble containing a reassortment of components, perhaps with the proteins that attach to a human cell but with other features that give it the virulence of the avian virus, including the ability to infect cells outside the respiratory tract. This reassortment of viral RNA segments in a cell infected by two strains of influenza virus (human and bird flu) may result in a new and potentially dangerous strain that could spread easily from human to human and so trigger a deadly worldwide epidemic. Such genetic mixing might occur in pigs, since a pig might be infected by both strains and then pass the new virus on to humans. Alternatively, a person might become infected with bird flu and human flu and start an epidemic of the novel virus.

Experts are in general agreement that there are very real reasons to worry that a potential H5N1 pandemic will have far greater impact than the 1918 Spanish flu:

1. The world is much more densely populated now than in 1918, and much more of today's population is concentrated in citites. Influenza (and other respiratory viruses) spreads wildly among dense populations.
2. The world is home to more elderly, chronically ill, and immuno-compromised people now than in 1918. These groups are at an increased risk of dying from flu.
3. The ease of air travel today increases the potential for viruses to spread across the globe quickly and broadly.
4. The H5N1 strain of today is far more deadly than its 1918 counterpart, which killed 2.5% of those it infected.

Research suggests that currently circulating strains of H5N1 viruses are becoming more capable of causing disease in animals than were earlier H5N1 viruses. One study found that ducks infected with H5N1 virus are now shedding more virus for longer periods without showing symptoms of illness. This finding has implications for the role of ducks in transmitting disease to other birds and possibly to humans as well. Additionally, other findings have documented H5N1 infection among pigs in China and H5N1 infection in felines (experimental infection in housecats in the Netherlands and isolation of H5N1 viruses in tigers and leopards in Thailand). In addition, in early March 2006, Germany reported H5N1 infection in a stone marten (a weasel-like mammal). The avian influenza A (H5N1) virus that emerged in Asia in 2003 continues to evolve and may adapt so that other mammals may be susceptible to infection as well.

The H5N1 in Asia and parts of Europe is not expected to diminish significantly in the short term. It is likely that H5N1 infection among birds has become endemic in certain areas and that human infections resulting from direct contact with infected poultry will continue to occur. So far, the spread of H5N1 virus from person-to-person has been rare and has not continued beyond one person. There is little pre-existing natural immunity to H5N1 infection in the human population. If these H5N1 viruses gain the ability for efficient and sustained transmission among humans, an influenza pandemic could result, with potentially high rates of illness and death.

Ten Things to Know About Pandemic — from The World Health Organization

1. <u>Pandemic influenza is different from avian influenza.</u> "Avian influenza" refers to a large group of different influenza viruses that primarily affect birds. On rare occasions, these bird viruses can infect other species, including pigs and humans. An influenza pandemic happens when a new subtype emerges that has not previously circulated in humans. Avian H5N1 is a strain with pandemic potential; once it adapts to the human host, it will no longer be a bird virus — it will be a human influenza virus.

2. <u>Influenza pandemics are recurring events.</u> An influenza pandemic is a rare but recurrent event. Three pandemics occurred in the previous century: "Spanish influenza" in 1918, "Asian influenza" in 1957, and "Hong Kong influenza" in 1968. A pandemic occurs when a new influenza virus emerges and starts spreading as easily as normal influenza – by coughing and sneezing. Because the virus is new, the human immune system will have no pre-existing immunity. This makes it likely that people who contract pandemic influenza will experience more serious disease than that caused by normal influenza.

3. <u>The world may be on the brink of another pandemic.</u> Health experts have been monitoring the H5N1 virus strain for nearly eight years, watching it kill 57% of the humans it infects. Presently, the virus does not jump easily from birds to humans or spread readily and sustainably among humans. However, should H5N1 evolve to a form as contagious as normal influenza, a pandemic could begin.

4. <u>All countries will be affected.</u> Once a fully contagious virus emerges, its global spread is considered inevitable. Countries might, through measures such as border closures and travel restrictions, delay arrival of the virus, but cannot stop it. Given the speed and volume of today's international air travel, the virus could spread very rapidly, possibly reaching all continents in less than 3 months.

5. <u>Widespread illness will occur.</u> Because most people will have no immunity to the pandemic virus, infection and illness rates are expected to be higher than during seasonal epidemics of normal influenza. Current projections for the next pandemic estimate that a substantial percentage of the world's population will require some form of medical care. Few countries have the staff, facilities, equipment, and hospital beds needed to cope with large numbers of people who suddenly fall ill.

6. <u>Medical supplies will be inadequate.</u> Supplies of vaccines and antiviral drugs – the two most important medical interventions for reducing illness and deaths during a pandemic – will be inadequate in all countries at the start of a pandemic and for many months thereafter. Inadequate supplies of vaccines are of particular concern, as vaccines are considered the first line of defense for protecting populations. On present trends, many developing countries will have no access to vaccines throughout the duration of a pandemic.

7. <u>Large numbers of deaths will occur.</u> To provide a useful and plausible planning target, WHO uses a conservative estimate that 2 million to 7.4 million deaths may occur. This estimate is based on the comparatively mild 1957 pandemic. If the virus is more virulent — closer to the one seen in 1918, death tolls will climb much higher.

(continued)

8. <u>Economic and social disruption will be great.</u> Past pandemics have spread globally in two and sometimes three waves. Not all parts of the world or of a single country are expected to be severely affected at the same time. Social and economic disruptions could be temporary, but may be amplified in today's closely interrelated and interdependent systems of trade and commerce. Social disruption may be greatest when rates of absenteeism impair essential services, such as power, transportation, and communications. High rates of illness and worker absenteeism are expected, and these will contribute to social and economic disruption.

9. <u>Every country must be prepared.</u> WHO has issued a series of recommended strategic actions, designed to provide nations of the world with different layers of defense that reflect the complexity of the evolving situation.

10. <u>WHO will alert the world when the pandemic threat increases.</u> WHO works closely with ministries of health and various public health organizations to support countries' surveillance of circulating influenza strains. A sensitive surveillance system with six distinct phases provides categories to the current threat. As of this writing, the threat is categorized as phase 3: a virus new to humans is causing infections, but does not spread easily from one person to another.

Pandemic <u>Will</u> Change Everyday Life

An especially severe influenza pandemic could lead to high levels of illness, death, social disruption, and economic loss. Everyday life would be disrupted because so many people in so many places become seriously ill at the same time. Pandemics typically have occurred in 2-3 waves, spanning the course of 12 to 24 months, so it is critical that you be prepared to ride out the likely sources of disruptions of daily life.

In a pandemic, everyday life as we know it will suddenly halt. In its place we may find that:

- Social disruption may be widespread
- Being able to work may be difficult or impossible
- Health care facilities, banks, stores, restaurants, government offices, and post offices, may be closed for an extended period of time
- Transportation services may be disrupted

Economic and social disruption will likely be widespread. Impacts can range from school and business closings to the interruption of basic services such as public transportation and food delivery. Travel bans, closings of schools and businesses and cancellations of events could have major impact on communities and citizens. People may choose to stay home to keep away from others who are sick, and people may need to stay home to care for ill family and loved ones, resulting in significant worker absenteeism.

According to the World Bank, even a flu with "normal" characteristics in terms of transmissibility and deadliness could have serious consequences for the global economy if the world's population has limited immunity. Presuming infection of some 35 percent of the population (as estimated by WHO in 2005), the World Bank projects that pandemic flu will result in a US $965.4 Billion cost to the world economy. Even though individuals are only temporarily unavailable from work, the impact on output here is more than twice as large as from the loss of life, because the affected population is so much large. In addition, people will go to extreme measures to avoid getting sick, resulting with a 20% decline in air travel, tourism, restaurant meals, and usage of mass transportation services. All totaled, the total impact of a shock combining all these elements is 3.1% for the global economy.

Preparedness is critical in preparing for pandemic, and communications and information are critical components of pandemic response. Each of us must take steps to educate ourselves on what a pandemic is, what needs to be done at all levels to prepare for pandemic influenza, and what could happen during a pandemic. Should a pandemic occur the public must be able to depend reliable, objective sources to provide scientifically sound public health information quickly, openly and dependably.

Relevant Websites for Information on Bird Flu

Infection Protection: Pandemic Avian Flu Update: www.worldhealth.net/pandemic

The World Health Network, the official website of the A4M and the Internet's leading anti-aging portal: www.worldhealth.net

MyLongLife.com, an informational website on the subject of human longevity: www.mylonglife.com

U.S. Department of Health & Human Services Avian Influenza website: www.pandemicflu.gov

U.S. Centers for Disease Control & Prevention Avian Influenza webarea: http://www.cdc.gov/flu/avian/index.htm

World Health Organization Avian Influenza webarea: http://www.who.int/csr/disease/avian_influenza/en/index.html

---

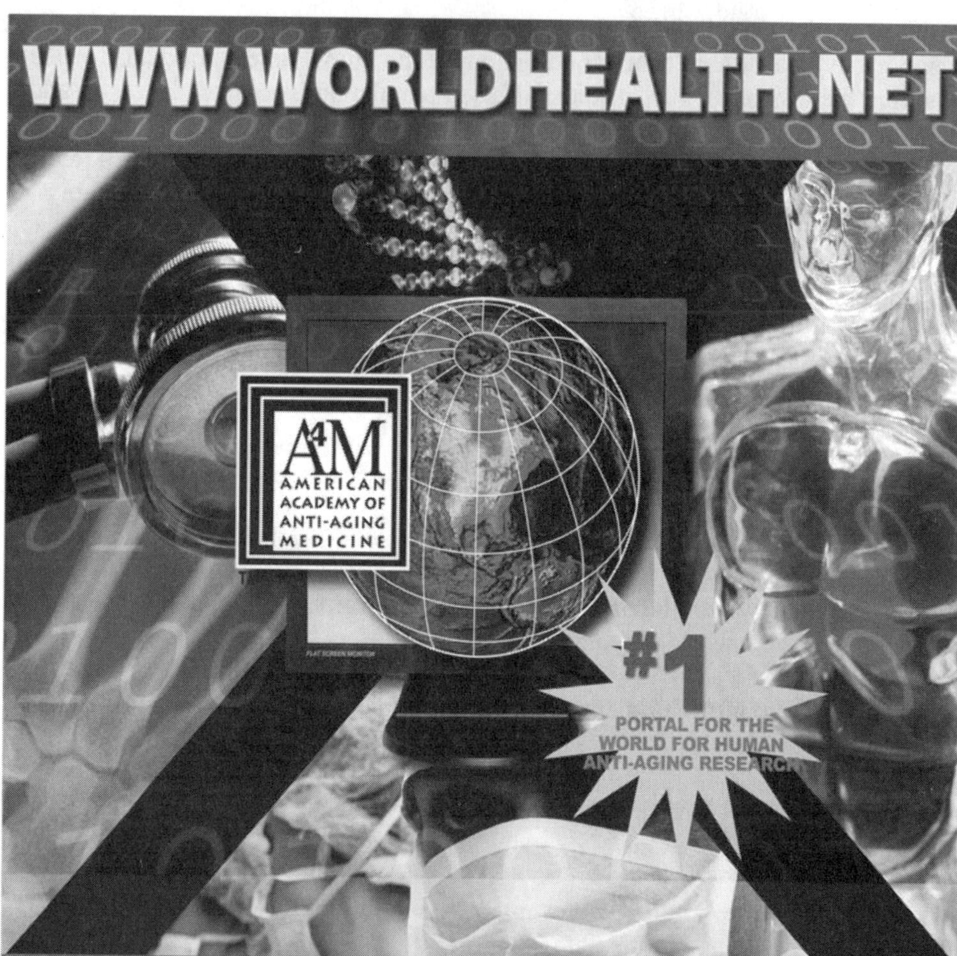

WWW.WORLDHEALTH.NET
A4M
AMERICAN ACADEMY OF ANTI-AGING MEDICINE
#1
PORTAL FOR THE WORLD FOR HUMAN ANTI-AGING RESEARCH
• Listed #1 For Anti-aging Related Keywords On Google, Yahoo, MSN, AOL And Other Major Search Engines.
• 20 Million Hits Per Month
• FREE Electronic Bio-Newsletter ($149 Value)
• World's Leading Resource Of Anti-Aging Related News
• Online Video Directory Of Physicians, Products And Services
• Archival Library Of Over 100,000 Referenced Research Papers
WWW.WORLDHEALTH.NET

Chapter 2. Medical Overview

Introduction to the Flu

What Is the Influenza Virus?

Influenza is a highly contagious viral respiratory infection of the upper respiratory tract. The virus that causes the flu enters the body's airways through mucous membranes in the nose, eyes, or mouth. Once the flu infection invades the body, it can settle into the throat, nose, bronchial tubes, lungs, and middle ear, causing an array of discomforting symptoms.

Influenza can be spread widely and wildly due to the fact that it can be transmitted from person-to-person by coughs and sneezes. It is estimated that a single sneeze can project up to 4,500 viral droplets, moving at speeds up to 100 miles per hour. If someone with the flu in your immediate proximity (3-4 feet [1-1.2 meters]) sneezes, you can become exposed and catch it. Good hygiene habits, including proper and frequent handwashing (see Chapter 3), are of the utmost importance in reducing one's risk of contracting the flu.

There are three types of influenza viruses, designated types A, B, and C. Influenza virus A is a genus of a family of viruses called Orthomyxoviridae in virus classification. Influenza virus A has only one species in it; that species is called "Influenza A virus". Variants of this species are sometimes named according to the species the strain is endemic in or adapted to, namely: human flu, bird flu, swine, flu, horse flu, and dog flu.

"Human influenza virus" usually refers to those subtypes that spread widely among humans. Influenza A virus is subdivided into subtypes based on hemagglutinin (H) and neuraminidase (N) protein spikes from the central virus core. There are 16 H types, each with up to 9 N subtypes, yielding a potential for 144 different H and N combinations. As of this writing, H1N1, H1N2, and H3N2 are the only known Influenza A virus subtypes currently circulating among humans.

The annual flu (also called "seasonal flu" or "human flu") in the U.S. results in approximately 36,000 deaths and more than 200,000 hospitalizations each year. In addition to this human toll, influenza is annually responsible for a total cost of over $10 billion to the U.S. economy. Not only deadly, influenza compromises health, leaving people more susceptible to pneumonia, ear infections, and sinus difficulties.

Symptoms of Seasonal Flu

Both the common cold and seasonal flu cause upper respiratory symptoms. Both of these maladies begin similarly, with body aches, cough, fatigue, headache, and hot and cold sweats. However, with the flu, it is common for a fever to develop, along with a dry throat and cough. In addition, nausea and vomiting may occur. The seasonal flu can last up to 12 days or more, followed by a week or more of residual coughing and fatigue.

The following chart outlines symptoms that differentiate these two maladies apart from each other:

Characteristic	Seasonal Flu	Common Cold
Pathogen	Orthomyxoviridae	Rhinovirus
Chest congestion	Common and can become severe. Pneumonia is also a common complication.	Common, but mild to moderate
Cough	Common and can be severe	Hacking
Fever	Usually high (102-104°F [38.8-40°C]). May last 3-4 days.	Rare (except in young children)
Chills	Common and can be severe	Mild or none
General aches and pains	Usual and can be severe	Mild
Headache	Common	Rare
Sneezing and/or red, watery, itchy eyes.	Common	Rare
Sneezing	Occasional	Usual
Sore throat	Occasional	Usual
Stuffy nose	Occasional	Usual
Tiredness	Severe	Mild
Nausea and vomiting	Occasional	Rare
Lingering fatigue	Common, can last 1-3 weeks	Mild if any.
Primary season	Winter months	Late August through April
Duration	Up to a month	7-10 days

The risk of an individual's susceptibility to flu increases with:
- Stress, excessive fatigue, and poor nutrition
- Recent illness that has lowered resistance
- Chronic lung or heart disease
- Pregnancy (3rd trimester)
- Living in close quarters to others
- Immunosuppression from drugs or illness
- Being in a crowded place when a flu epidemic occurs

Prevention of Seasonal Flu

Seasonal Flu Vaccine

The seasonal flu vaccine significantly narrows the chances of getting and transmitting the flu virus. It is highly recommended that high-risk groups receive the vaccine, such as:
- People at high risk for complications from the flu:
    - People 65 years and older
    - People who live in nursing homes and other long-term care facilities that house those with long-term illnesses
    - Adults and children 6 months and older with chronic heart or lung conditions, including asthma
    - Adults and children 6 months and older who needed regular medical care or were in a hospital during the previous year because of a metabolic disease (like diabetes), chronic kidney disease, or weakened immune system (including immune system problems caused by medicines or by infection with human immunodeficiency virus [HIV/AIDS])
- Children 6 months to 18 years of age who are on long-term aspirin therapy. (Children given aspirin while they have influenza are at risk of Reye syndrome.)
- Women who will be pregnant during the influenza season
- All children 6 to 23 months of age
- People with any condition that can compromise respiratory function or the handling of respiratory secretions (that is, a condition that makes it hard to breathe or swallow, such as brain injury or disease, spinal cord injuries, seizure disorders, or other nerve or muscle disorders.)
- People 50 to 64 years of age. Because nearly one-third of people 50 to 64 years of age in the United States have one or more medical conditions that place them at increased risk for serious flu complications, vaccination is recommended for all persons aged 50 to 64.
- People who can transmit flu to others at high risk for complications. Any person in close contact with someone in a high-risk group (see above) should get vaccinated. This includes all health-care workers, household contacts and out-of-home caregivers of children 6 to 23 months of age, and close contacts of people 65 years and older.

Flu viruses are constantly mutating (changing), so the composition of the seasonal flu vaccine is different each year. To battle the current year's version of the flu, experts at the World Health Organization, the U.S. Centers for Disease Control and Prevention, and the U.S. Food and Drug Administration collect and analyze those mutations and choose the three most likely viral suspects for the current year's vaccine. Consequently, the seasonal flu vaccine protects against only 2 or 3 specific strains of influenza A, and does not protect against the H5N1 bird flu virus.

When a person receives a flu vaccine by injection, the body creates antibodies, specialized immune agents that will attack the live virus(es) should they invade your system. It is uncommon for people to contract the flu from the flu shot itself—about 1% or less, according to experts. However, soreness in the arm receiving the vaccine, starting the next day and lasting for 1-2 days, is common.

Because it can take two weeks for the vaccine to provide full immunity, experts note the optimal period for administration of the flu vaccine is October 1 through November 15, preceding the winter months in which seasonal flu epidemics most often occur.

Seasonal Flu Vaccine Do's and Don'ts

- <u>DO</u> get a flu vaccine if you are traveling out of the country. Air travel puts you at high-risk for contracting the flu, since many people are in close proximity to each other and the passenger cabin often uses recirculated air. Also, consider that seasons are different outside this country (reversed for the Southern Hemisphere). In addition, getting sick in a developing nation without having a flu shot may put you at higher risk for its complications. See Strategy #10 in Chapter 3 for a more detailed discussion on tips to travel smart and safely.
- <u>DO NOT</u> get the seasonal flu vaccine if:
  - You have a severe allergy to chicken eggs
  - You have had a severe reaction to an influenza vaccination in the past
  - You have developed Guillain-Barré syndrome (GBS) within 6 weeks of getting an influenza vaccine previously
  - You have a moderate or severe illness with a fever (wait to get vaccinated until symptoms lessen)
  - Children less than 6 months of age (influenza vaccine is not approved for use in this age group)

2006-2007 Flu Vaccine Recommendations

The U.S. Centers for Disease Control & Prevention (CDC) is preparing for its broadest and most ambitious vaccination yet for the coming influenza season. The CDC expects to have 120 million doses of seasonal flu vaccine available, the most ever available to-date. Additionally, the CDC has extended its recommendations to include children aged up to 5 years and all their contacts (siblings, parents, and caregivers) to receive the vaccine; last year, only children age 6 months to 2 years were on the priority list.

Treatment of Seasonal Flu

Antibiotics are useless against all illnesses that are viral in nature, including influenza. Treatment is largely limited to alleviation of symptoms, with generally helpful measures such as:

- Relieving nasal congestion: Use saline (salt water) drops, 1 teaspoon of salt to 1 quart of water
- Relieve chest congestion: Inhale steam from a pan of boiled water for 15 minutes every 2-4 hours; or take a long hot shower
- Relieving sore throat: In 8-ounces (236 mL) of warm water, dissolve 2 aspirin tablets (325 mg each) and 1 teaspoon (5 ccs) of salt. Gargle for 5 minutes and spit it out (do not drink it).
- Mobilizing lung secretions: Use an ultrasonic, cool-mist humidifier and drink warm teas and water.
- Coughing up mucous secretions: Splint ribs with a towel, then lean over the toilet with your head-down; cough to release excess mucous secretions from your nose and mouth.
- Getting plenty of bedrest to minimize aches and pains.
- Staying hydrated: Drink 8 ounces (236 mL) of water every hour while awake (more if you have a fever), in which you have added 2 tablespoons (30 ccs) of freshly squeezed lemon juice (for added flavonoids and to help alkalinize [see "Immunity Desk Reference" in Chapter 3] the body).
- Avoiding sugary fruits (oranges and bananas) and carbohydrate-laden grains and pastas, which are foods that viruses feed on to survive.

When medication is needed, antiviral drugs (oseltamivir [Tamiflu] or zanamivir [Relenza]) can be administered. (We discuss these two medications in further detail in Chapter 4, in the context of their potential use for bird flu.) To treat seasonal flu, however, these antiviral drugs must be started within the first 48 hours after symptoms start. This narrow window of opportunity is often too short, for many people do not realize they have contracted the flu within the first 48 hours. Neither Tamiflu nor Relenza cure the flu, but rather help to alleviate symptoms and shorten the duration of illness.

A Bird's Eye View of Bird Flu

Why the Concern?

The H5N1 virus is one of 16 different known subtypes of avian influenza (bird flu) viruses. H5N1 viruses have been found in birds around the world. The virus can infect chickens, turkeys, pheasants, quail, ducks, geese, and guinea fowl, as well as a wide variety of other birds, including migratory waterfowl. As the spread of H5N1 infection among birds increases, so does the opportunity for H5N1 to be transmitted directly from birds to humans. When an influenza virus "jumps" species from an animal, such as a chicken, to infect a human, the result is usually a "dead-end" infection that cannot easily spread further in the human population. However, mutations in the virus could develop that allow efficient human-to-human transmission.

If avian and human influenza viruses were to simultaneously infect a person or animal, the two viruses might swap genes. The result could be a new virus that is readily transmissible between humans and against which humans would have no natural immunity. Such an event could trigger a worldwide influenza pandemic.

Health professionals are concerned that the continued spread of a highly pathogenic avian H5N1 virus across eastern Asia and other countries represents a significant threat to human health. The H5N1 virus has raised concerns about a potential human pandemic because:

- It is especially virulent
- It spreads via migratory birds
- It can be transmitted from birds to mammals and in some limited circumstances to humans
- Like other influenza viruses, it continues to evolve

Outbreaks of avian influenza H5N1 occurred among poultry in eight countries in Asia (Cambodia, China, Indonesia, Japan, Laos, South Korea, Thailand, and Vietnam) during late 2003 and early 2004. At that time, more than 100 million birds in the affected countries either died from the disease or were killed in order to try to control the outbreaks. By March 2004, the outbreak was reported to be under control.

Beginning in June 2004, however, new outbreaks of influenza H5N1 among poultry and wild birds were reported in Asia. Since that time, the virus has spread geographically. Reports of H5N1 infection in wild birds in Europe began in mid-2005. In early 2006, influenza A H5N1 infection in wild birds and poultry were reported in Africa and the Near East.

Remarks Michael Leavitt, Secretary, U.S. Department of Health & Human Services (HHS) "It is only a matter of time before we discover H5N1 in birds in America. The migration patterns of the wild fowl that carry the virus make its appearance here almost inevitable." Any of the migratory birds that fly over North America can, once infected, then carry the virus hundreds — or thousands — of miles across the nation in any direction:

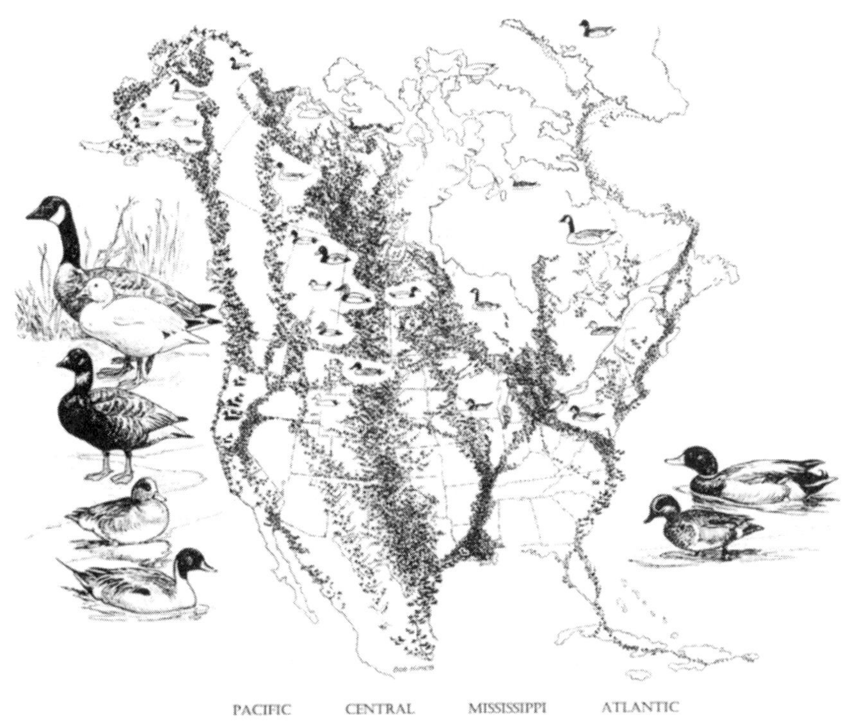

Waterfowl Flyways of North America

Image credit U.S. Forestry & Wildlife Service.
Image from www.pandemicflu.gov, U.S. Department of Health & Human Services, accessed 9 May 2006.

Since 2003, a growing number of human H5N1 cases have been reported in Azerbaijan, Cambodia, China, Djibouti, Egypt, Indonesia, Iraq, Thailand, Turkey, and Vietnam. <u>More than half of the people infected with the H5N1 virus have died.</u> Most of these cases are all believed to have been caused by exposure to infected poultry. There has been no sustained human-to-human transmission of the disease, but the concern is that H5N1 will evolve into a virus capable of human-to-human transmission.

Slow but Steady Progress in Beating H5N1 in Asia

As of May 2006, Vietnam — where almost 50 percent of the initial cases were reported — has not reported a single human case or an outbreak of flu in poultry this year. This lack of outbreak is attributed to massive-scale vaccination of the poultry whereby all of the nation's 220 million chickens were vaccinated.

Thailand — the second-hardest-hit nation — has also not seen a human case for over a year and a poultry outbreak for since late 2005. The nation culled affected birds and compensated farmers who lost their poultry stock. Thailand has also vaccinated its fighting cocks, a large source of gaming revenue and favorite sport among locals. In addition, Thailand has appointed a volunteer deputy in every village whose responsibility it is to report sick chickens to officials.

Both Vietnam and Thailand did not hold back supplies of Tamiflu, the anti-viral drug of choice for treatment of bird flu (see Chapter 4). These supplies were sent to even the smallest regional hospitals and health workers were ordered to begin treating suspected cases even if confirming diagnosis was still pending.

Another possible success case is China, where the Chinese Agriculture Ministry appears to have delivered on its promise to vaccinate all domestic poultry. The number of reported human cases in China have been low over the last two years. So far in 2006, China reported only 10 cases as compared to 8 for the same timeframe in 2005. "We are hopeful that China has turned the corner," remarked Dr. David Nabarro, chief pandemic flu coordinator for the United Nations.

"Tomorrow, the whole thing could change again," says Dr. David Nabarro. "We need to be on the alert at all times."

What is the Avian Flu?

Avian influenza — aka "bird flu" — is an infection caused by influenza viruses that occur naturally in birds. There are different subtypes of these viruses because of changes in certain proteins (hemagglutinin [HA] and neuraminidase [NA]) on the surface of the influenza A virus and the way the proteins combine. Each combination represents a different subtype denoted by the identification code H#N#.

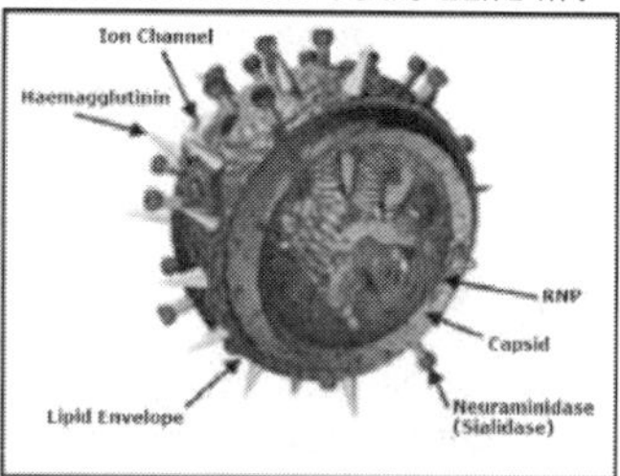

The H5N1 virus molecule is characterized by the proteins Hemaggluttinin (HA) and Neuraminidase (NA)

Image from "Pandemic Planning Update," U.S. Department of Health & Human Services, 13 March 2006, http://www.pandemicflu.gov/plan/pdf/panflu20060313.pdf. Accessed 9 May 2006.

Prominent Bird Flu Virus Subtypes

All known subtypes of influenza A viruses can be found in birds. There are 16 known HA subtypes and 9 known NA subtypes of influenza A viruses. Avian influenza A H5 and H7 viruses can be distinguished as "low pathogenic" and "high pathogenic" forms on the basis of genetic features of the virus and the severity of the illness they cause in poultry; influenza H9 virus has been identified only in a "low pathogenicity" form. Each of these three avian influenza A viruses (named for the hemagglutinin [HA] protein, as H5, H7, or H9) theoretically can be partnered with any one of nine neuraminidase [NA] surface proteins, yielding potentially nine different forms of each subtype (e.g., H5N1, H5N2, H5N3, H5N9 etc.).

Influenza A H5
- Potentially nine different subtypes
- Can be highly pathogenic or low pathogenic
- H5 infections have been documented among humans, sometimes causing severe illness and death

Influenza A H7
- Potentially nine different subtypes
- Can be highly pathogenic or low pathogenic
- H7 infection in humans is rare, but can occur among persons who have direct contact with infected birds; symptoms may include conjunctivitis and/or upper respiratory symptoms

Influenza A H9
- Potentially nine different subtypes
- Documented only in low pathogenic form
- At least three H9 infections in humans have been confirmed to-date

---

E-Biotech Newsletter

Information on the Latest in Advancements in Human Longevity — Including Immune Health Delivered to Your Desktop
An Educational Service of The World Health Network
FREE SUBSCRIPTIONS ($149 value)! Sign up at **www.worldhealth.net**

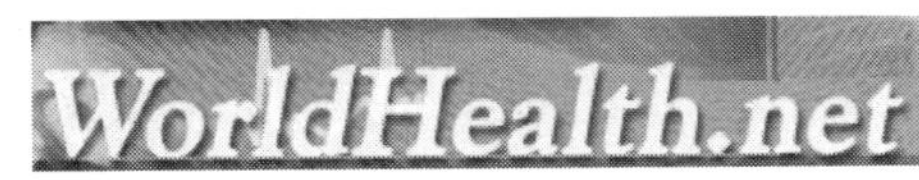

Expert Insight: We are "sitting ducks" because "we do so much wrong in this country"

Dr. John B. Symes ("DogtorJ.") is a practicing veterinarian who, following his personal diagnosis of celiac disease (gluten intolerance) and subsequent recovery from numerous chronic ailments, has become an Internet medical researcher and consultant (www.dogtorj.net). The following is an excerpt from an interview conducted by Dr. Ronald Klatz with Dr. Symes; you are invited to visit www.worldhealth.net/pandemic to listen to the entire interview.

Dr. Ronald Klatz: [W]hat everyone seems to be concerned about right now, is the looming pandemic that our government tells us could possibly kill 2 million Americans and may be 150 million people worldwide and I just want to get your take on that, because after all you are veterinary researcher and this is bird flu. The disease is afflicting primarily fowl, not humans, even though, I believe the human death toll is over 200 right now. The fowl death toll is in the hundreds of millions, may be you can go into that a little bit.

Dr. John Symes: Well, fortunately it is still outside our borders, but we have been reading about it. I have not been seeing a lot in the veterinary literature. To be honest … our biggest concern is in the feline. The cat is susceptible to the H5N1 virus and they have had some actually died and had a number of them experimentally infected — even big cats, some of the leopards and tigers and some of the smaller exotic cats like civets are all susceptible to this, so the feline population is the one that we are most concerned about. There was a study done that showed that out of 600 dogs or something that were studied, a quarter of them were at least having antibodies to the Avian influenza virus, but no known clinical disease in the dog.

So, for the small animal practitioner the biggest concern will be the cat and there have been some cats reported died of the disease especially experimentally. They not only will shed the virus from the respiratory tract, but actually in their feces apparently. But, at this point, the amount of virus that they are shedding appears to be low, so they don't think that will be a major contributing factor to the spread of the disease. The main way that these cats are acquiring the virus is through the feeding or eating of raw bird carcasses because cooking fortunately does a good job of destroying this, but eating raw carcasses is the big concern. So, we see a lot of interspecies spread of these viruses. The dog, in this country, we recently had an upper respiratory virus that came from the horse and started infecting the dog. We note that these things move around, but our biggest concern is going to be the cat.

RK: Dr. Symes, what is your read on this? Do you think that the H5N1 is going to mutate into something that is going to affect people and is that concerning the veterinary community, is there any preparation going on the veterinary community?

JS: Most people have demonized viruses completely and they feel like that viruses only do bad things, but of course as you and I know viruses are essential to the operation of

(continued)

Expert Insight with Dr. Symes *(continued)*

nature and the two things that they do most that are good is they allow adaptation and they also cause variation in nature. Viruses are ubiquitous in all aspects of nature plants, animals, and humans. We are loaded up with them and that is because they help us to adapt to this ever changing environment. From the moment the world was created, it has never been the same and the viruses are in this mix to help us adapt to this ever changing environment and so when we talk about viruses mutating, if we look at it just purely that way we have a tendency, you know, to think it is just something bad. All of a sudden this [benign virus] turns out into [a malignant virusl and goes and starts killing millions of people when sometimes it happens like it did back in 1918, but the main thing is that they adapt and they are forced into adaptation because they are going to survive; that is one of the things, they are like a little robot, they are going to survive that is what their charge is and they are going to adapt and allow whatever there are living in to survive and until the adaptation process gets to the point where it has to become pathogenic to survive. So, the development of pathogenic viruses, the way I look at it my perspective is that they simply have been forced into adapting to something that our bodies no longer like because they are going to survive no matter what.

The reason why they are concerned about millions and millions of people dying in this country from this kind of thing if you were ever to do that and become the next Spanish flu is because we do so much wrong in this country with our diet and our life style and our lack of sleep and our abuses of alcohol, drugs and cigarettes and everything else and all lack of hygiene as well.

We have got to start the best preparation if we knew this thing [bird flu] is going to hit us in 10 to 15 years later on 100th-year anniversary of Spanish flu or something we would have to make a major turnaround in just how we live our lives, mainly on diet and lifestyle, that is to me the only true prevention because our immune systems and the shape that they are in right now, we are sitting ducks.

Visit www.worldhealth.net/pandemic to listen to the entire interview with Dr. Symes

---

Avian Influenza in Birds

Avian influenza is an infection caused by avian (bird) influenza (flu) viruses. These influenza viruses occur naturally among birds. Wild birds worldwide carry the viruses in their intestines, but usually do not get sick from them. However, avian influenza is very contagious among birds and can make some domesticated birds, including chickens, ducks, and turkeys, very sick and kill them.

Infected birds shed influenza virus in their saliva, nasal secretions, and feces. Domesticated birds may become infected with avian influenza virus through direct contact with infected waterfowl or other infected poultry, or through contact with surfaces (such as dirt or cages) or materials (such as water or feed) that have been contaminated with the virus.

Infection with avian influenza viruses in domestic poultry causes two main forms of disease that are distinguished by low and high extremes of virulence. The "low pathogenic" form may go undetected and usually causes only mild symptoms (such as ruffled feathers and a drop in egg production). However, the highly pathogenic form spreads more rapidly through flocks of poultry. This form may cause disease that affects multiple internal organs and has a mortality rate that can reach 90-100% often within 48 hours.

Influenza A (H5N1) virus – also called "H5N1 virus" – is an influenza A virus subtype that occurs mainly in birds, is highly contagious among birds, and can be deadly to them. H5N1 is the strain of avian flu currently of concern for potential pandemic outbreak in humans. H5N1 virus does not usually infect people, but infections with these viruses have occurred in humans. Most of these cases have resulted from people having direct or close contact with H5N1-infected poultry or H5N1-contaminated surfaces.

Avian Flu in Birds is On the Rise

- Wild birds can carry the viruses, but usually do not get sick from them. However, some domesticated birds, including chickens, ducks, and turkeys, can become infected, often fatally if they come into contact with an infected wild bird. Domesticated birds usually die from the disease.
- The H5N1 virus is endemic in much of Asia and has now spread into Europe. Avian H5N1 infections have recently killed poultry and other birds in a number of countries.
- Strains of avian H5N1 influenza may infect various types of animals, including wild birds, pigs, and tigers.
- Symptoms in birds and other animals vary, but virulent strains can cause death within a few days.

Human Infection with Avian Influenza Viruses

"Human influenza virus" usually refers to those subtypes that spread widely among humans. As of this writing, there are only three known A subtypes of influenza viruses (H1N1, H1N2, and H3N2) currently circulating among humans. All known subtypes of influenza A viruses can be found in birds. It is likely that some genetic parts of current human influenza A viruses originally came from birds. Influenza A viruses are constantly changing, and other strains might adapt over time to infect and spread among humans.

The risk from avian influenza is generally low to most people, because the viruses do not usually infect humans. H5N1 is one of the few avian influenza viruses to have crossed the species barrier to infect humans, and it is the most deadly of those that have crossed the barrier.

Usually, "avian influenza virus" refers to influenza A viruses found chiefly in birds, but infections with these viruses can occur in humans. Although avian influenza A viruses usually do not infect humans, more than 200 confirmed cases of human infection with avian influenza viruses have been reported since 1997. Most cases of H5N1 influenza infection in humans have resulted from contact with infected poultry (such as, domesticated chicken, ducks, and turkeys) or surfaces contaminated with secretion/excretions from infected birds.

Because of concerns about the potential for more widespread infection in the human population, public health authorities closely monitor outbreaks of human illness associated with avian influenza. To date, human infections with avian influenza A viruses detected since 1997 have not resulted in sustained human-to-human transmission. So far, the spread of H5N1 virus from person to person has been limited and has not continued beyond one person. Researchers from the University of Wisconsin's School of Veterinary Medicine (USA) found that the receptors favored by the H5N1 virus are located deep within the lower respiratory tract — primarily on cells of the alveoli and some in the bronchi — suggesting that the unimpeded transmission of H5N1 may require the ability of the virus to recognize yet-unrecognized human flu receptors. Nevertheless, because all influenza viruses have the ability to change, scientists are concerned that H5N1 virus one day could be able to infect humans (perhaps by recognizing the receptors deep in the lungs) and then spread easily from one person to another.

In the current outbreaks in Asia, Europe, and Africa, more than half of those infected with the H5N1 virus have died. Most cases have occurred in previously healthy children and young adults. However, it is possible that the only cases currently being reported are those in the most severely ill people, and that the full range of illness caused by the H5N1 virus has not yet been defined.

Why So Deadly?

The H5N1 virus is highly effective at replication. After invading its first host cell, the virus takes over so much of the cell's machinery that the cell dies. The virus then ejects itself to new, live host cells, one by one, to repeat the process again and again. An accumulation of dead cells in the airways results in a runny nose and scratchy throat. Too many dead cells in the lungs result in death.

Contrary to the commonly held belief that the bird flu virus has little affinity for human respiratory tissues, a researcher team from Erasmus Medical Center (Netherlands) has found that the H5N1 virus readily attaches to, and proliferates, within the bronchioles and alveoli of the human lungs. The team notes that this preference by the virus for cells in the deepest passageways of lung tissue "may contribute to the severity of the pulmonary lesion [caused by bird flu infection]."

Because these viruses do not commonly infect humans, there is little or no immune protection against them in the human population. If H5N1 virus were to gain the capacity to spread easily from person to person, a pandemic (worldwide outbreak of disease) could begin. No one can predict when a pandemic might occur. However, experts from around the world are watching the H5N1 situation very closely and are preparing for the possibility that the virus may begin to spread more easily and widely from person to person.

Symptoms of Bird Flu in Humans
Symptoms of bird flu in humans range in severity and may include:
- Typical human influenza-like symptoms, including:
  — Fever: temperature over 100.4°F (38°C)
  — Cough
  — Sore throat
  — Muscle aches
- Early symptoms may include diarrhea, vomiting, abdominal pain, chest pain, and bleeding from the nose and gums (watery diarrhea without blood appears to be more common in H5N1 avian influenza than in normal seasonal influenza)
- Eye infections (conjunctivitis)
- Pneumonia
- Severe respiratory diseases (such as acute respiratory distress)
- Viral pneumonia
- Other severe and life-threatening complications

Infection and Transmission
The U.S. federal government has made these assumptions about pandemic flu:
- Persons who become ill may shed virus and can transmit infection for up to one day before the onset of illness. Viral shedding and the risk of transmission will be greatest during the first 2 days of illness. Children usually shed the greatest amount of virus and therefore are likely to pose the greatest risk for transmission.
- On average, infected persons will transmit infection to approximately two other people.

Progression of the Disease
The World Health Organization (WHO) has made these observations regarding the progression of the disease in affected individuals:
- Time between onset of illness to the development of acute respiratory distress can range between 4 to 13 days — 6 days is typical. Some severe cases have been observed to arrive at respiratory failure 3 to 5 days after symptom onset.
- Difficulty in breathing develops around five days following the first symptoms. Respiratory distress, a hoarse voice, and a crackling sound when inhaling are commonly seen. Sputum production is variable and sometimes bloody.
- Abnormal lab tests commonly include: leukopenia (mainly lymphopenia), mild-to-moderate thrombocytopenia, elevated aminotransferases, and, in some instances — disseminated intravascular coagulation.
- Almost all patients develop pneumonia. Multiorgan dysfunction is common. Pneumonia and/or multiorgan dysfunction cause death.

Differentiating Bird Flu from Seasonal Influenza

Unlike seasonal influenza, in which infection usually causes only mild respiratory symptoms in most people, H5N1 infection may follow an unusually aggressive clinical course, with rapid deterioration and high fatality. Primary viral pneumonia and multi-organ failure have been common among people who have become ill with H5N1 influenza.

Seasonal (or common) flu is a respiratory illness that can be transmitted person to person. Most people have some immunity, and a vaccine is available. More information about seasonal influenza is available from the US Centers for Disease Control & Prevention, at http://www.cdc.gov/flu/.

Avian (or bird) flu is caused by influenza viruses that occur naturally among wild birds. The H5N1 variant is deadly to domestic fowl and can be transmitted from birds to humans. There is no human immunity and no vaccine is available.

IMPORTANT: The influenza vaccine administered for the 2005-06 season does not provide protection against avian influenza. The seasonal flu vaccine contains two strains of the most recent form of influenza A as well as one strain of influenza B. These strains have widely circulated in humans for a number of years. The vaccine for bird flu being tested is made with an inactivated H5N1 virus that approximates the strain of avian flu anticipated to affect humans (see Chapter 4 for the discussion on Bird FluVaccine).

Expert Insight: "Brain washed with the idea of immunity"

Mr. Fintan Dunne is a technical and medical journalist and editor of MyLongLife.com (www.mylonglife.com). He has written on medical issues as diverse as HIV/AIDS, SARS, and the social psychology of medicine. The following is an excerpt from an interview conducted by Dr. Ronald Klatz with Mr. Dunne; you are invited to visit www.worldhealth.net/pandemic to listen to the entire interview.

Dr. Ronald Klatz: Tell us about the scientific process involved in identifying the bird flu virus organism.

Mr. Fintan Dunne: If you want to prove the existence of a new pathogenic strain, you should ideally isolate it in sufficient titre (in other words in sufficient quantity) from an animal or person suspected to have it. From that you should be able to grow it in-culture, you should be able to centrifuge it, and you should be able to find significant numbers of similar multigenic (similar size, similar shape) — to indicate you have isolated something. Then you can take that something — still unproven as to effect — inject it into another animal or person, and it should achieve the same symptoms as in the first person or animal. It's a long time since we've done that, and we don't — believe it or not — do it with HIV AIDS. Of course it is difficult: you cannot potentially inject somebody with something which is going to cause AIDS, but surprising we are not doing that kind of stuff in things like SARS and bird flu, but we are making inferences based on antibody responses and we are relying on technology such as for example PCR which is a DNA or RNA amplification techniques.

(continued)

Expert Insight with Mr. Fintan Dunne *(continued)*

Now you can amplify for that does improve sufficient titre, but that they might been something there which is disease causing and seeing sufficient titre or not could be indicative of a problem.

RK: Fintan, you are saying that we have not isolated this specific organism that causes bird flu that all these things of dead chickens and other fowl or no body has gone so far to take tissue samples from them and isolate out an organism?

FD: Isolation can done in individual instances where you're attempting to prove that such and such causes a disease. The problem is that when it goes on to doing the kind of testing which we rely on to determine whether it is an epidemic or not. We are not using that. We are using indirect markers, which are basically the culpability of hemagglutinin — so we're inferring that hemagglutinin in influenza virus — we're inferring. The H5N1 stands for hemagglutinin N5 and neuraminidase N1. And this is in theoretical construct, I'm afraid. If you look at possible causes for what we see, the pattern is that we're not seeing the spread in wild birds as was projected, we're not seeing this H5N1 to any degree as the so-called outbreak in mass production poultry facilities (if you look there, the key issue there may be the levels of selenium which the birds have, selenium is very important in its antiviral effect within the animal and human body, and selenium is becoming deficient in these birds). We're also looking at so-called human cases associated with these. After these case are taking place against a backdrop of 3.5 million upper respiratory tract infections, which are taking place around the globe annually. So to isolate out small set of the 5, 6, 7, or 10 here there. Unfortunately, that the cases we are dealing with within realms of the normal error risk of any procedure. So you can't inference from these isolated cases. We saw this in SARS where Dr. Frank Plummer in Canada, with Toronto being one of the epicenters of SARS, was finding that these so called coronavirus, which was the alleged cause of this syndrome was in at first 40% of the patients that were suspected, then 30%, then 20%. In other words, 80% of the people that were hospitalized and suspected of SARS were suffering just from influenza and there we have no proof that coronavirus was actually the cause. I think it is a growing symptom that it's the terrain — underlying substrate — in the susceptibility of an individual towards these tendencies.

RK: So you are saying, if, my understanding is correct, you are saying that we have not or the established medical authorities have not proven an isolatable specific organism for either SARS nor for avian flu.

FD: The problem arises because we have been brain washed with this idea of immunity. It is very controversial issue in relation to vaccination, but the idea is that antibody immunity confers protection. We know from there have been various campaigns which have been conducted to vaccinate, but we have had epidemics among the vaccinated (which don't seem

(continued)

Expert Insight with Mr. Fintan Dunne *(continued)*

to differentiate whether they've been vaccinated or not), and so antibody immunity is a bit of a misnomer. And so indeed, there is this whole idea of a small set of external viruses which come after us and get us. For example, in the case of HIV there is clear evidence that 95% actually have the genetic sequence of HIV endogenously within the cells and that this only emerges and becomes active in particular when the selenium levels are low or in response to toxic assaults or the overall nutritional condition of metabolic condition of the body. So, we are very focused on this idea of external agents, but we have a multiple mess of animal and human viral bits of pieces in there in what they call the junk DNA section of our DNA. In many cases we have taken a superfluous route that everything in the body is perfect and everything that comes from outside is a threat and so we developed this whole rationale and we see all these epidemics in that light. But if we look at them and we know that in fact it is those who have compromised health — on the one hand we think that there are germs out there which will come and get you, it doesn't matter if you're a quarterback in perfect physical health, it will take you down — but at the same time we do accept that the aged and the younger are the ones most at-risk when there's any kind of an epidemic. I suggest that it's the health of an individual that is the key in all of this.

RK: Okay. Well, I certainly can accept that but I have a hard time getting that we are dealing with a phantom when it comes with when it comes like avian flu, certainly with all the government prepared. The TV specials, the World Health Organization leafleting everybody at the airports; in US alone $7 Billion has been earmarked for preparedness for the avian flu epidemic that is supposed to come any day.   There is even talk of special quarantine areas they want to initiate... What is behind all this stuff?
FD: Well, there is an agenda. The agenda is to a degree, a conscious agenda to say, the conscious agenda is to continue with this that there is external agents which can take you down with regard to health status, which is incredibly simplistic, but it does serve to bolster the weak position — growing weaker by the day — of the entire pharmaceutical/corporate complex based around this notion of disease. So it suits that agenda. There are suspicions behind this agenda as well, to demonize the small owner, who has small stocks of animals, at the expense of large production units, and then following hysteria about the bird flu epidemic to begin to make the claim that only large production units could possibly have the safety standards to make sure that never happens again. But that's the world of politics, so leave that to them … there's a lot of politics in health.

Visit www.worldhealth.net/pandemic to listen to the entire interview with Mr. Dunne

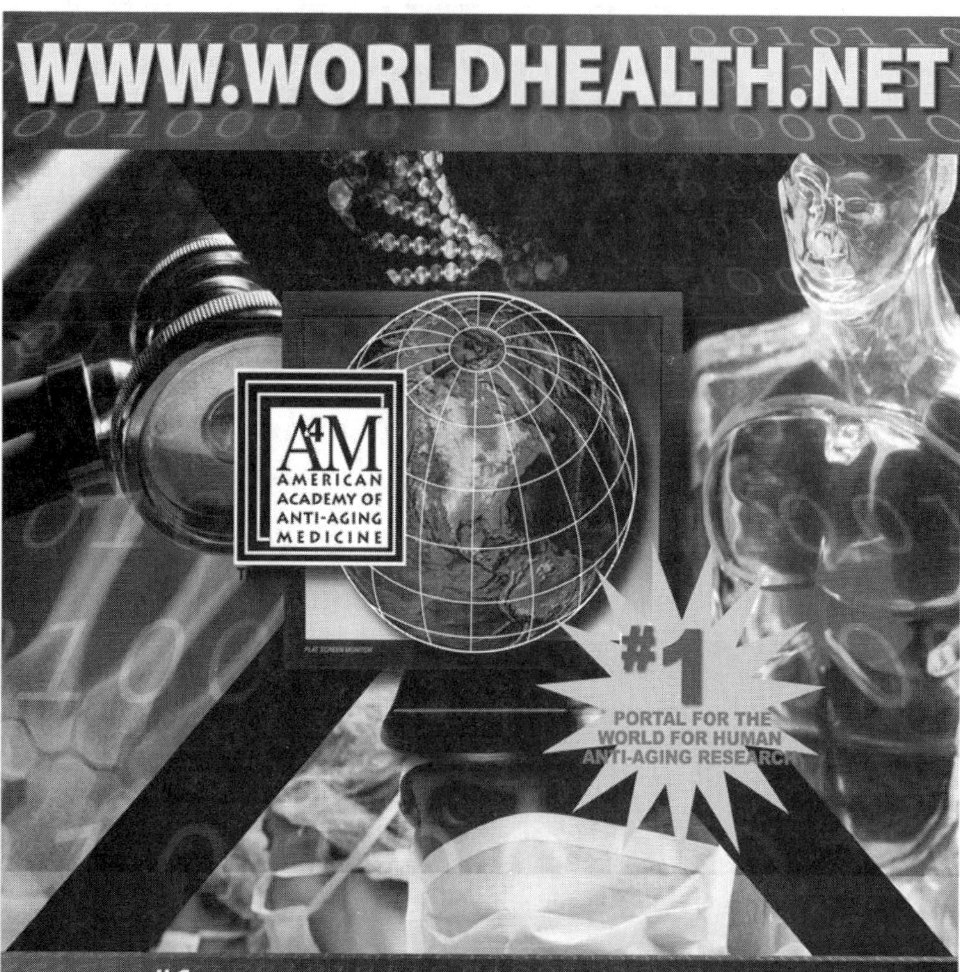
WWW.WORLDHEALTH.NET
A4M
AMERICAN ACADEMY OF ANTI-AGING MEDICINE
#1
PORTAL FOR THE WORLD FOR HUMAN ANTI-AGING RESEARCH
• Listed #1 For Anti-aging Related Keywords On Google, Yahoo, MSN, AOL And Other Major Search Engines.
• 20 Million Hits Per Month
• FREE Electronic Bio-Newsletter ($149 Value)
• World's Leading Resource Of Anti-Aging Related News
• Online Video Directory Of Physicians, Products And Services
• Archival Library Of Over 100,000 Referenced Research Papers
WWW.WORLDHEALTH.NET

Chapter 3. Top Ten Preventive Strategies for Optimizing Immune Function

Introduction

In this chapter we present the Top Ten strategies that aim to help you to optimize the performance of your immune system, as well as enhance your overall immune resistance to a wide variety of infectious diseases. The strategies are:

Strategy #1. Hygiene habits
Strategy #2. Natural immune enhancement
Strategy #3. Hydration
Strategy #4. Daily nutrition
Strategy #5. Poultry safety
Strategy #6. Face masks and respirators
Strategy #7. Barriers
Strategy #8. Ventilation
Strategy #9. Humidification
Strategy #10. Travel tips

By deploying these ten Strategies as a unified effort, you improve your body's ability to ward off a wide variety of infectious pathogens. Be mindful, however, that these Strategies are not in any way to be considered as specific preventive or treatment approaches for avian flu in-specific, or influenza in-general. Selection and deployment of an appropriate immune-optimizing strategy for your specific personal needs should be done only with the advisement of a qualified physician or health practitioner.

First, we preface these ten strategies with a discussion on the bird flu vaccine presently in-development, which serves to underscore the importance of these Top Ten strategies.

Discussion on the Bird Flu Vaccine

Vaccination is one of the most effective ways to minimize suffering and death from influenza. Influenza vaccines are given as a preventive measure to elicit a protective immune response in the body. When immunized, the body is poised to remember this virus and can better fight an infection caused by it.

However, there is currently no vaccine available to protect humans against the H5N1 virus. Clinical trials of a vaccine are underway, but whether or not the studies conclude before the coming of bird flu to U.S. soil is uncertain.   To complicate matters, a pandemic vaccine cannot be produced until a new pandemic influenza virus emerges and is identified, so the vaccine being tested today may not be the one that is effective against the particular strain of H5N1 that will arrive in the United States. Additionally, production and supply shortages may plague the ability for the vast majority of Americans to procure vaccination. And just recently, vaccines – including those for influenza – have been found to be less effective as we age.

The Vaccine Development Track: A Shot in the Dark?

Experts speculate that the first global wave of illness is expected to be over before enough vaccine specific to the pandemic strain has been made, and by then the virus could well mutate into yet another different strain. According to the U.S. Department of Health & Human Services (HHS): "There likely will be no vaccine initially available that precisely matches the pandemic strain when a pandemic begins. Because influenza viruses continually evolve and mutate, it is not possible to develop a vaccine until after the pandemic strain actually comes into existence. Only after the strain emerges, is isolated and characterized can a vaccine be developed and manufactured. Based upon current vaccine production processes and capacities, it will take at least 6 months to begin producing pandemic vaccine once a pandemic strain occurs."

Vaccine development efforts in the United States are now underway. As part of the U.S. federal plan to prepare for pandemic, on 4 May 2006 the U.S. HHS awarded more than $1 billion to five companies, to accelerate development and production of new technologies for influenza vaccines within the U.S. This is in addition to a previous $97 million contract aimed to develop a cell-based vaccine on a commercial scale.

Research studies to test a vaccine to protect humans against H5N1 virus began in April 2005, when The National Institute of Allergy and Infectious Diseases (NIAID), initiated fast-track recruitment for a Phase I clinical trial to investigate the safety of a vaccine against H5N1 avian influenza in 451 healthy adults ages 18 to 64. This clinical trial aims to establish the safety of the H5N1 vaccine and its ability to generate an immune response (immunogenicity). Based on preliminary data from 117 of the 450 participants enrolled in the trial in healthy adults, two 90-μg doses of the H5N1 candidate vaccine generated the highest immune response among those doses tested. Further clinical testing is underway, including the evaluation of techniques that may reduce the amount of antigen (active ingredient) per dose needed to achieve effective individual protection. A full report from the trial is pending.

A similar trial of the vaccine in persons 65 and older, which began in October 2005, has completed recruitment. A third similar trial, in children ages 2 through 9 years old, opened in January 2006 and has also completed recruitment. No reports from these two trials are yet available.

<u>Early tests indicate the vaccine currently under development is effective in only 50% of patients. It also requires a dose 12-times stronger than a regular annual flu shot. Two shots are also required.</u>

Vaccine Concerns: A Shot of False Hope?

Mutation of the Virus

If the H5N1 virus currently circulating mutates considerably before the vaccine is ready for the public, it is unknown whether it will still be effective. Flu viruses change over time (a process known as "antigenic drift"). However, in response to the increasing number of H5 cases reported in early 2004, public health officials deemed it critical to move ahead quickly and select one of the available human H5 viruses for vaccine production. The clinical trials taking place in 2005 and 2006 evaluate an inactivated vaccine made from an H5N1 virus isolated in Southeast Asia in 2004. The H5N1 reference virus (the strain used to produce the H5N1 vaccines for NIAID's clinical trials) was developed by researchers at St. Jude Children's Research Hospital (Memphis, TN USA) using a technique known as reverse genetics.

If a distinct H5N1 virus should suddenly emerge, an additional new vaccine against that strain may be needed. Public health officials are banking on the fact that "the experience gained by manufacturers in producing the current H5N1 vaccine should make us better prepared for the next time."

Production & Supply Shortages

Stretching the Vaccine Supply

In a study published in May 2006, researchers discovered that a theoretical way to extend the quantity and effectiveness of a vaccine — by adding chemicals called adjuvants — failed for the H5N1 vaccine. The adjuvant studied actually lessened the effectiveness of the smallest dose of H5N1 vaccine. Disappointed experts instead encourage focus on the matter of global manufacturing capacity as a leading priority.

Most of us vividly recall the shortage of seasonal influenza vaccine that occurred in the fall of 2004. In October of that year, Chiron Corporation notified U.S. federal health officials that its influenza vaccine (Fluvirin) would not be available for distribution in the United States for the 2004-05 influenza season. The company indicated that the Medicines and Healthcare Products Regulatory Agency in the United Kingdom, where Chiron's Fluvirin vaccine is produced, suspended the company's license to manufacture Fluvirin vaccine in its Liverpool facility, thereby preventing any release of this vaccine for the influenza season. The result was a reduction by approximately one-half the expected supply of trivalent inactivated vaccine (flu shot) available in the United States for the 2004-05 influenza season. Vaccinations were limited to administration to only select subpopulations: children under 2 years of age, seniors over age 65, pregnant women, and persons with chronic medical conditions ages 2 to 64. Healthy men and women were expressly prohibited from receiving the vaccination. Yet, at the end of the 2004-05 influenza season, hospitals, nursing homes, and private medical offices had an excess of the vaccine on-hand, and were forced to discard tens of thousands of doses.

The U.S. federal government learned an important lesson from the Chiron supply stoppage, namely that it needed to institute mechanisms to promote greater diversification of the U.S. influenza vaccine supply. In a statement by Jesse L. Goodman, M.D., M.P.H. Director, Center for Biologics Evaluation and Research before The Committee on Government Reform in February 2005, he observed that "[W]ith an adequate vaccine supply supplemented by effective antivirals we can greatly decrease our vulnerability and provide protection against influenza. FDA [The U.S. Food & Drug Administration] recognizes the need to work with multiple partners, including manufacturers, to increase supply and to support progress toward more modern, dependable methods of production."

In this same testimonial statement, Goodman announced plans by the federal government to prepare to respond effectively to the next influenza pandemic. Contracts were awarded in an effort to move the United States from dependence solely on egg-based production technology for vaccines, to the development of domestically-produced U.S. licensed cell-culture based and/or recombinant protein and DNA-based vaccines. It is hoped that moving from an egg-based production to a cell-culture production can potentially shorten the time needed to produce vaccine as well as decrease the risk of contamination inherent in egg-based production. In addition, studies supported by the U.S. National Institutes of Health (NIH) and FDA aim to develop vaccine strategies that could lead to longer lived immunity and to vaccines that help protect against multiple strains of influenza. Hopes Goodman: "Through all these efforts, and with enhanced global surveillance by CDC and its partners, we have the unique opportunity to effectively intervene and potentially blunt a global pandemic, should one occur."

HHS plans to stockpile this experimental "pre-pandemic" H5N1 vaccine, with the expectation that it may offer some level of immune protection should the H5N1 virus mutate into a pandemic strain. There are, however, two potentially major pitfalls with this plan:

1. The stockpile consists of doses adequate to vaccinate up to 20 million people. As this book went to press, the United States was home to 299,000,534 residents. In an interview with "Dateline NBC" that aired on 23 April 2006, U.S. HHS Secretary Michael Leavitt commented that: "It will take three to five years for us to develop the manufacturing capacity to produce the 300 million courses of a vaccine necessary to treat the entire American public."

2. A vaccine must have specificity for the virus for which it is aimed to prevent. Being "close" is not enough. Being effective against a current virus strain, and not against its new, more virulent strain that emerges in the future, makes a vaccine useless.

Vaccines Are Less Effective as We Age

At the Ninth Annual Vaccine Research Conference, organized by the National Foundation for Infectious Diseases that took place in May 2006, University of California at Los Angeles (UCLA) professor Rita Effros, Ph.D. presented evidence showing that as we age, T cells (lymphocytes, the white blood cells that initiate the immune response) have reduced levels of CD28, a cell-signaling molecule key to mounting an immune response to vaccines. As a result, the incidence and severity of viral infections — including influenza — has been on the rise in the elderly, who are at particularly high-risk of having extremely low CD28 levels. Lone Simosen, Ph.D., of the U.S. National Institutes of Health, speculated that: "The absence of a decline in national influenza-related mortality rates since 1980 could be due to a suboptimal vaccine effect ...."

Expert Insight: It's like "living in New Orleans" — wondering if those levees are going to fail

Mark Blatter, MD, is Medical Director of Primary Physicians Research, Inc., located in Pittsburgh, Pennsylvania. Dr. Blatter is also clinical Instructor at Children's Hospital of Pittsburgh; Clinical Associate Professor of Pediatrics, Department of Pediatrics, University of Pittsburgh School of Medicine; and is in private practice at Pediatric Alliance, St. Clair, in Pittsburgh. Dr. Blatter is also a vaccinologist, having investigative experience that includes more than 130 clinical trials in 20 years. The following is an excerpt from an interview conducted by Dr. Ronald Klatz with Dr. Blatter; you are invited to visit www.worldhealth.net/pandemic to listen to the entire interview.

Dr. Ronald Klatz: We are looking for answers with regard to how real and significant is the current concern that avian flu will infect humans and that they will lead to mass causalities, and what can be done about this. Even beyond that, if we forget the concerns coming from the CDC and the World Health Organization — they are talking about millions and millions of people dead worldwide, may be as many as a 150 million. Forgetting all that if we just look at influenza in the United States every year, we are looking at about 36,000 to 37,000 people who die from that alone. So, just good old garden-variety influenza is a [mass] killer. God forbid that a worldwide pandemic occurs. So, what's your take overall to the concerns that the media has been playing about this risk of new infectious agents.

Dr. Mark Blatter: The question has not been a matter of, "if" we are going to have to spread to humans, but just a matter of "when" we will have to spread to humans. I think that what people need to realize is, it's a same kind of view that the people who used to live in New Orleans had, where every year we would always worry about "Boy I wonder if those levees are really going to work? But yeah, they have been working well for so long, why we should we worry about it now it's not going to happen." But we found out unfortunately that it wasn't the case. So, this is a matter of major public concern.

(continued)

Expert Insight with Dr. Mark Blatter *(continued)*

RK: What I am shocked to find is the position is that, [most] everyone [in government and the media] is waving red flags and saying, "be afraid, be very afraid, worry, worry, worry. This is a real risk." We have got to do something about it, but there is very little in the way of clinical guidelines on how to treat this condition and what to do. Have you seen anything in that regard [that can protect us]?

MB: In work that was done on the new vaccine, one of the vaccines that is being worked on right now, on the one hand, they said they found it encouraging that 50% of the patients responded to the vaccine. Well, one could say that is pretty good, but for any other vaccines we use, we generally take a guideline of at least upper 70s or higher percentage response to consider it to really be a success. Normally for most adults, anyone who has had flu vaccine in the past, all you need is one dose of vaccine, and as you saw, even with the shortages we had in recent winter, just even getting one dose into every person, that is a huge lines at clinics all around the country. Now, what you have to realize is in the trials that we have just done. They had to give two doses a month apart. So, think about what happened before and now think about that being doubled.

Now, the other problem that also exists is they had to use somewhere between 3 and 6 times the amount of antigen in the vaccine that is normally used in a regular flu vaccine. You are going to be able to make much less vaccine because you have to use so much more per shot and you are giving two shots to people. So again, it is going to be very difficult to make enough vaccine to supply the entire population. The bottom line of it is, there are no good guidelines right now because we do not know what the eventual face of this disease will look like.

RK: Well, that's another issue isn't it that we don't even have a vaccine to H5N1 because the vaccines that have been produced are not going to be effective against the eventual bug that mutates that is going to cause human-to-human transmission.

MB: Well, we don't know that for a fact. It is always a possibility that might but right now the odds are it won't. But if we can go ahead and make a vaccine that is effective, and by the way, when I mentioned before about the vaccines not being overly effective, that was without an adjuvant. An adjuvant is something that's added to a vaccine, to kind of boost up the immune response that our body has to the vaccine. If the vaccines that are being used so far are adjuvanted, then the hope is that you will get a better response. They will be more effective.

When we talk what will eventually happen that if we go ahead and say that, on a normal flu season, as a general average, we generally have about 40,000 deaths, what you said upper30s, and about 200,000 people hospitalized every year from influenza which in itself is horrible, and it is indictment of the system of medical care in this country. That we have not been pushing a relatively inexpensive solution to the problem by just having universal flu shots, everyone being immunized, but if in the best case scenario, as the people

(continued)

Expert Insight with Dr. Mark Blatter *(continued)*

were saying when the [avian flu] virus makes the mutation that allows it to start spreading human-to-human, it generally becomes less virulent. Now, the best case scenario is if it becomes a lot less virulent. The best case scenario that we will jump from 40,000 deaths to about 200,000 deaths and that the hospitalizations will jump from about 200,000 to about a million but that's the best case scenario.

What has been keeping people awake at night for now a number of years, is the worst case scenario and the numbers that we have been talking about, this is just United States, this is not the world. In just the United States, if the worst case ever happened, and it does not significantly change its virulence, we are talking about close to 1.9 to 2 million people dead and many many many millions of people will need to be hospitalized in a society that will not have enough hospitals, enough beds or enough healthy doctors or nurses to care for [all the patients].

RK: What about newer methods for vaccine production? I believe that we are still using technology that's dozens if not decades old right now. What about the newer technologies that we are supposed turn out vaccines in a matter of weeks?

MB: Right now, we are still using chicken and eggs. The limiting factor is always going to be a proper supply of chickens and eggs. But in reality, there are new techniques, self-cultured techniques and other techniques that may allow us to respond in a period of months, still a month or two rather than the four or five that it might take right now to produce vaccine. But again, let's remember that when this jump occurs, and when we start to know that we have got a major problem, the likelihood that we will have much around for the first month or two or three as this disease starts to spread is not likely.

[Bird flu] will affect a much greater segment of our society and at this time, it will not respect race, gender, what party you have voted for or your degree of affluence because this time, it will affect everyone.

RK: What is it that an individual can do for themselves?

MB: The bottom line is, as an individual, you can do nothing. However, [I urge you to] get your routine flu shots not because that will help you for the flu pandemic, but just because it is the right thing to do to make sure you stay healthy. Next point is, good health practices, and by that I mean just doing the right things. If you are healthy, you are more likely to survive anything whether it be, heart disease, diabetes, or a stroke. You are much more likely to survive if you are not overweight, and not smoking, and you are exercising, and you are eating healthy. So, that is what you should be doing. Finally, we all should be praying for: milder disease as the virus evolves; more antiviral availability; and pray for possible breakthroughs in rapid vaccine manufacture.

Visit www.worldhealth.net/pandemic to listen to the entire interview with Dr. Blatter

> **Protect Yourself and Your Family**
>
> The government expects vaccination of fewer than 1 in 10 Americans to help delay or lessen the initial impact of a pandemic, while a vaccine against the actual pandemic strain is developed and produced. Additionally, vaccines have now been found to be less effective as we age.
>
> Take the matter of protecting you and your family into your own hands. Start you natural immune-optimizing regimen today (see "Immunity Desk Reference" in Strategy #2 below), and prepare for the worst (see Chapter 5).

Strategy #1. Hygiene Habits

In the case of prevention from contracting the H5N1 virus, "back to basics" seems to be the rule:

- Wash your hands frequently and properly.
- Cover your mouth and nose when you cough or sneeze. Use a tissue, a paper towel, your shirtsleeve — anything in lieu of sneezing into the open air (especially in a confined space such as a plane or office setting, where other people are in close proximity).
- Promptly discard used tissues in a wastebasket.
- Clean your hands after coughing or sneezing. Use soap and water or an alcohol-based hand cleaner.
- Avoid people who are sick. Stay at home if you are sick.

Above all, the most effective way to promote your body resistance to invasion by pathogenic germs of any kind, is to practice healthy hygiene habits — the most critical of which is proper and frequent handwashing.

Handwashing

Professor John Oxford of Queen Mary's School of Medicine (London, United Kingdom) has warned that: "Unfortunately, personal cleanliness and hygiene levels have dropped steadily over the last decades with many microbes, as never before, using the opportunity to spread." He suggests: "First and foremost to reduce virus transmission, attention must be paid to handwashing and then when this is satisfactory, focus on cleansing surfaces and equipment shared by others such as desks, tables, telephone, and door knobs."

Viruses can survive on human hands for several hours and then can be spread by direct contact. As well as through coughs and sneezes, an individual may pick up the virus on their fingers by touching an infected object or person. If that person then rubs their nose or eyes with their contaminated fingers they can become ill and spread the infection to others. Typically, germ counts on the hands of the general population range as follows:

	Male	**Female**
Thumbnail	50-900 million	350,000-650,000
Index nail	800,000-1.1 million	850,000-17 million
Other fingernails	100-1.2 million	250,000-700,000
Palm	100-4,700	450-2.1 million
Back of hand	4000-1,000	25-200
Counts are per square centimeter (about the surface area of a shirt button).		

Exchange Sentiments, Not Germs
Long considered customary politenesses upon meeting someone, handshaking and cheek-kissing are also prime ways that viruses can readily transmit from person-to-person. Consider other options for greeting a friend, such as:
- Nod your head
- Bow
- Bump knuckles
- Bear (side-by-side) hug

In the event you do receive someone's handshake or cheek-kiss (despite your best efforts to avoid doing so), immediately proceed to the restroom and wash your hands and face.

The best defense to protect against a virus — be it H5N1, the seasonal influenza bug, or other — is simple: keep your hands clean by washing them properly and frequently.

Penny Wise
Washing hands regularly costs less than a penny, which can prevent a $50 or more office visit to the doctor to merely diagnose an infectious disease you contract.

Wash your hands ten times each day — double that if you're in an environment where infectious germs abound (for example, proximity to someone sick in the home or at the workplace, or physical contact with objects touched by someone who is sick). It is especially important to wash hands:
- Before, during, and after you prepare food (particularly raw meat, poultry, or fish)
- Before you eat
- Before inserting or removing contact lenses
- After you use the bathroom
- After you blow your nose, cough, or sneeze
- After treating a cut or wound of your own or someone else
- After handling animals or animal waste
- After changing a diaper
- After handling garbage

- When your hands are visibly dirty
- More frequently when you or someone in your home is sick

The U.S. Centers for Disease Control & Prevention (CDC) outlines the technique for proper handwashing as:

1. Wet your hands and apply liquid or clean bar soap. Place the bar soap on a rack that allows it to drain.
1. Scrub all surfaces — including wrists, palms, backs of hands, fingers, under the fingernails, and between fingers. Rub your hands vigorously together for 10-15 seconds.
3. Rinse well with warm water.
4. Dry hands with a clean or disposable towel. Pat the skin rather than rubbing, to avoid chapping or cracking. Apply hand lotion if your skin is susceptible to drying out.

By definition, soap contains compounds that dissolve the lipid (fat)-bearing parts of a virus molecule, rendering it noninfectious. Any brand of soap will do, but antibacterial soaps are more active against certain bacteria and spores that can cause other diseases.

Perhaps just as important as washing your hands is the matter of properly drying them. Researchers at Auckland Hospital in New Zealand found that rinsed but undried hands can transfer tens of thousands of bacterial cells to food. Their follow-up studies found that drying hands for ten seconds using a clean cloth towel followed by air drying for 20 seconds achieved a 99.8% reduction in the amount of bacteria moved from one place to another on the skin. The same technique also reduced the bacteria moved from human hands to food by 94%.

Don't Spread the Wealth (of Germs)
- A fresh paper towel is preferred to a cloth that is damp or has not been laundered recently.
- Wiping damp hands on clothes or hair can spread bacteria to other areas of the body.

Make A Graceful Exit
In a public setting, perhaps as important as proper handwashing is how you exit the restroom itself. It is problematic, from a germ-avoidance perspective, that restroom doors often open inward. To avoid recontamination by the same microorganisms you so diligently removed from your hands:
- Use a clean, dry paper towel to grab doorknobs or pull doors open, and discard the towel promptly
- Use a pen or paperclip to hook the door handle and pull it open
- Open doors with your elbows or feet, which are areas of the body less prone to spreading infectious disease.

When running water is not available or readily accessible, in lieu of handwashing cleanse with an alcohol-based hand sanitizer (follow product instructions).

Personal Space Safety

Be careful of how close you get to others. Viruses — including the flu — can tranmit from person-to-person through handshakes and kisses. A sneeze or cough can propel a virus 10 or more feet (3 or more meters). Cigarette smoke also spreads respiratory viruses, so it's a good idea to avoid coming into contact with a smoke plume.

According to the U.S. Implementation Plan for the National Strategy for Pandemic Influenza, released 3 May 2006: "Human influenza virus is transmitted from person-to-person primarily via virus-laden large droplets (particles >5 µm in diameter) that are generated when infected persons cough, sneeze, or speak. These large droplets can then be directly deposited onto the mucosal surfaces of the upper respiratory tract of susceptible persons who are near (i.e., typically within 3 feet [1 meter] of) the droplet source. Transmission also may occur through direct and indirect contact with infectious respiratory secretions."

The Implementation Plan specifies the following infection control measures to reduce virus transmission:

<u>Persons who are potentially infectious should:</u>

- Stay home if they are ill
- Cover their nose and mouth when coughing or sneezing
- Use facial tissues to contain respiratory secretions and dispose of them in a waste container
- Wash their hands (with soap and water, an alcohol-based hand rub, or antiseptic handwash) after having contact with respiratory secretions and contaminated objects/materials (hand hygiene).

<u>Persons who are around individuals with influenza-like symptoms should:</u>

- Maintain spatial separation of at least 3 feet (1 meter) from that individual
- Turn their head away from direct coughs or sneezes
- Wash their hands (with soap and water, alcohol-based hand rub, or antiseptic handwash) after having contact with respiratory secretions and contaminated objects/materials.

Disinfection

The influenza virus is very contagious, and can remain on hard surfaces for up to 72 hours. Even after 72 hours, enough virus particles can remain to potentially sicken people.

The Hot Zone

Microbiologist Charles Gerba of the University of Arizona warns of favorite hideout spots for bacteria and viruses:

- The average desk harbors 400 more times bacteria than the average toilet seat. "Keyboards are a lunch counter for germs."
- "[Bathroom] sinks ... have got everything bacteria likes. It's wet, it's moist. In a home we usually find more *E. coli* in a sink than a toilet."
- "Usually the dirtiest handles in public restrooms are urinal flush handles [in men's restrooms]."

Popular Germ Hangouts

Among the germiest places in the workplace:

	In the home:
— Phone receiver (25,127 germs per square inch)	— Kitchen sponge (7.2 billion germs per square inch)
— Desktop (20,961)	— Kitchen sink
— Computer keyboard (3,295)	— Toilet bowl
— Computer mouse (1,676)	— Kitchen garbage can
— Fax machine (301)	— Refrigerator
— Photocopy machine (69)	— Bathroom doorknob
— Toilet seat (49)	— Cutting board

The adage "Necessity is the mother of invention" may be your best tactic in keeping surfaces germ-free. For example, to reduce the need to touch the doorknob itself:

1. Tape the latch on doors open;
2. Tie a nylon cord to both sides of the doorknob, allowing sufficient slack between the two ends to provide a loop that can be easily grasped

Or, pull your sleeves over your hands when touching doorknobs and other surfaces on which germs are found and thrive.

Most importantly of all: Keep a supply of disposable antiseptic towelettes, and a wastebasket, near all phones, computers, fax machines, copiers, etc. Use a towelette each time prior to, and after, touching these items, and discard it promptly.

To kill influenza germs, clean and disinfect surfaces that may have become contaminated with flu secretions, using products that are EPA registered disinfectants. Use Lysol, household bleach, or similar disinfectants such as 3% hydrogen peroxide (follow product instructions) (In times of emergency, use a spray bottle to conserve your disinfectant supplies.)

The World Health Network
www.worldhealth.net
The Official Website of the American Academy of Anti-Aging Medicine (A4M)
The Internet's Leading Anti-Aging Portal

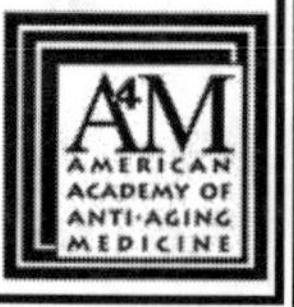

Strategy #2. Natural Immune Enhancement

The primary aim of this Strategy is to enhance and optimize an individual's overall immunity in an effort to minimize the adverse effects of exposure to any infectious pathogen. In the case of H5N1, we cannot count on vaccine to protect us (see the discussion earlier in this chapter), and we know that there will not initially be sufficient vaccine to inoculate everyone. Consequently, consider incorporating immune-enhancing nutritional supplements — in the form of vitamins, minerals, amino acids, and herbs; and natural immune-stimulating procedures, into your personal, advance preventive program for immune optimization.

<table>
<tr><td>

Buyer Beware

The U.S. Food and Drug Administration (FDA) has issued warnings to companies marketing bogus flu products, making unsubstantiated and unsupported claims that such products could be effective against preventing the bird flu or other forms of influenza.

Prior to purchasing a natural product purported to enhance immunity, look into the credibility and integrity of the company that manufactures or sells the product. Find out the company's history and track record. Reliable sources at which you may find assistance with this assessment are:

- The office of the Better Business Bureau for the city in which the company is located
- The web sites of the FDA (www.fda.gov) and FTC (www.ftc.gov)
- Determine (either by calling the company, or by reviewing their website):
  1. Is the company backed by legitimate, notable and published physicians and scientists who are not ashamed to have their names and credentials associated with the product?
  2. Is the company willing to furnish you with solid scientific research about its product? Have their findings been published in reputable scientific publications?
  3. Will the company provide you with the list of the specific ingredients in their product?

If the answer to any of these questions is "no," find an alternative source for the product.

For nutritional supplements, it is critical that you research the company(ies) from which you choose to purchase nutritional supplements, to be certain they are using pharmaceutical-grade ingredients and are GMP (Good Manufacturing Practices) Certified.

Consumers who believe they have seen a fraudulent product can report it to the FDA at: http://www.fda.gov/oc/buyonline/buyonlineform.htm

</td></tr>
</table>

> **Never Too Soon**
> Check with your anti-aging physician to create an immune optimizing regimen that is best suited for your specific needs. If nutritional supplements are part of your program, start taking them as soon as possible, certainly prior to a pandemic outbreak. Many nutritional supplements need days — sometimes weeks — to achieve optimal uptake and circulation in the body.

Introduction to the Human Immune System

Who Am I?

Immunocompetence, which is the body's biological sense of what is self and what is not, develops in the womb and in the first few months after birth. In the fetus, stem cells produced by bone marrow are called to "boot camp" in the thymus gland, where they develop into T-cells. The T-cells graduate if they learn how to recognize "self" by reading a unique molecular code that appears on the surface of all the cells in the body; if not, they are eliminated. This activity is part of a process called histocompatability—a term you are likely to hear more of as organ transplant technology evolves.

A healthy immune system captures and destroys things in the body that shouldn't be there—bacteria, viruses, parasites, chemicals, even splinters. Invaders that stay outside the cells are easier to conquer than those that enter cells. White blood cells are a key component of the immune system.   A cubic millimeter (cc mm) of blood normally contains 4,000 to 10,000 white blood cells. The ideal "white count" is about 6,000 to 7,000 per cubic mm of blood. Too few white blood cells means your immune response is low; too many means that your immune system is working inefficiently. Knowing the type of white blood cell that is elevated signals what kind of infection you have—bacterial, viral, or parasitic.

Battle Strategy

A nonspecific reaction is the immune system's most basic tactical move. When you cut yourself and the area swells and turns hot and pink, you're experiencing the symptoms of a nonspecific reaction. The more researchers study this initial reaction, the more they appreciate its complexity and importance.

Neutrophils, a type of white blood cell that patrols the body at all times, are the first to arrive at the trouble site. Neutrophils send distress signals and blockade the area so the infectious agent can't spread.

Macrophages, cells stationed at strategic points all over the body, are next on the scene. They start chewing up the invader and send out chemical messengers called cytokines that activate still more immune cells. Macrophages also prepare a rap sheet on the invader, packaging little pieces of the culprit as evidence for the helper T-cells that arrive later to assess the threat and plan a larger attack.

When a foreign element enters a cell, the cell itself has the ability to summon T-cells to the site. If the invader doesn't match the unique molecular code on the outside of the cell—that indicator of "self" discussed earlier—the T-cells will destroy it and will make new T-cells programmed to always remember that particular invader. This immunological memory is the power behind vaccines.

The immune system's special forces, white blood cells called *lymphocytes or T-cells and B-cells,* are part of what is called the learned or combinatorial immune system. They can slice and dice, shuffle and combine a limited number of genes to make tens of millions of antibodies and killer T-cells in response to specific invaders. While even the most primitive creatures have an immune system, it appears that only jawed vertebrates have the more advanced combinatorial system as well, the reason for which scientists still don't know.

Like neutrophils, lymphocytes originate from stem cells in the bone marrow. Some mature in the bone marrow and become B-cells, which produce and secrete antibodies. B-cells remain on alert in the lymphatic system until they are called into action.

Other lymphocytes become T-cells during a stay in the thymus gland. They circulate through the lymphatic system – a network of vessels, ducts and nodes that includes organs such as the tonsils, adenoids, spleen and appendix. The lymphatic system, which removes bacteria, viruses, antigens and other biowaste from circulation, is one of the body's three circulatory systems (the other two are the veins and the arteries). The lymphatic system connects to every organ in the body except the brain. The lymphatic system goes into high gear during infection and the lymph nodes nearest the infection become swollen with the filtered "non-self" microbes and biowaste from the infection itself.

There are several different kinds of T-cells, each with a specific duty:

- *Helper T-cells* dispatch and coordinate other T-cells and direct B-cells to make antibodies. Helper T-cells can live a long time and remember the invaders they've encountered. They can help . the immune system to react even faster in a repeat attack.
    - Some helper T-cells (TH1) deal with the immune response to bacteria, viruses and parasites; others (TH2) focus on allergic reactions and antibody responses. Research indicates that poor diet, high stress and exposure to environmental toxins can suppress TH1 activity. It's the nature of the system that when TH1 activity decreases, TH2 activity is increased. When this happens, TH2 cells secrete chronically high amounts of compounds that stimulate inflammation and fever. This reaction, when stimulated inappropriately or chronically, leads to inflammatory diseases such as arthritis and autoimmune conditions such as asthma, lupus, multiple sclerosis and chronic fatigue.
- *Killer T-cells (also called NK, or natural killer, cells)* have special receptors on their surface that recognize certain antigens, or invaders. When a cell is infected with a virus, for example, the cell presents a fragment of the virus on its surface. The killer T-cell latches on to this fragment, recognizes it as

"non-self" and injects a chemical called a cytokine into the cell to destroy the virus.

- Killer T- cells are the kamikazes of the lymphocyte army. All NK cells demonstrate an ability to inject a lethal substance to cause the cell to explode.
- *Suppressor T-cells* are the immune system's "cease fire" switch, keeping B cells and helper T-cells under control.
- Like killer T-cells, *B-cells* focus on only one antigen, bind with the antigen and morphing into large plasma cells that produce antibodies called immunoglobulins. These immunoglobulins patrol the body like smart bombs looking for their targets. Antibodies that respond to the first exposure to an antigen are very different from antibodies that cause an immediate allergic reaction.

The *thymus gland*, located in the chest, is a primary organ of the immune system. It activates T-cells and produces hormones key to the immune system. At puberty, our immune system reaches its zenith, and our thymus gland is at its largest. The thymus begins to shrink until by age 40 it is a shriveled shadow of its former self. By age 70, more than 95% of it has turned to fat or fibrous tissue. The shrinking thymus correlates with a rise in the diseases associated with aging, including cancer, autoimmune diseases, and infectious diseases. There is also a decline in T-cells and immune factors such as interleukin 2. As such, scientists believe that restoring thymus gland function can rejuvenate the immune system.

The thymus produces T-lymphocytes, essential for resistance to infection from mold-like bacteria, yeast (including Candida albicans), fungi, parasites, and viruses; and protection against development of cancer and autoimmune disorders including allergies and rheumatoid arthritis.

The thymus gland also releases hormones (thymosin, thymopoietin, and serum thymic factor), low levels of which are associated with depressed immunity and increased susceptibility to infection. Typically, thymic hormone levels will be very low in the elderly, individuals prone to infection, cancer and AIDS patients, and when an individual is exposed to excess stress.

The American Academy of Anti-Aging Medicine's (A4M) *Immunity Desk Reference*
IMPORTANT – PLEASE READ

The content presented in the American Academy of Anti-Aging Medicine's (A4M) *Immunity Desk Reference* is for educational purposes only. It is not intended to prevent, diagnose, treat or cure disease or illness. A4M's *Immunity Desk Reference* is not intended to provide medical advice, and is not to be used as a substitute for advice from a physician or health practitioner. Prior to engaging in any of the programs or therapies described in the A4M's *Immunity Desk Reference*, consult a knowledgeable physician or health practitioner.

While potentially therapeutic pharmaceuticals, nutraceuticals (dietary supplementation) and interventive therapies are described in the A4M's *Immunity Desk Reference*, this work serves the sole purpose of functioning as an informational resource. Under no circumstances is the reader to construe endorsement by A4M of any specific companies or products. Quite to the contrary, *Caveat Emptor*. It is the reader's responsibility to investigate the product, the vendor, and the product information.

The entries appearing in the *Immunity Desk Reference* are for consideration in optimizing an individual's overall immune function. They are not in any way to be considered as specific preventive or treatment approaches for avian flu in-specific, or influenza in-general. Selection and deployment of an appropriate immune-optimizing strategy for your specific personal needs should be done only with the advisement of a qualified physician or health practitioner.

Dosing of nutraceuticals can be highly variable. Proper dosing is based on parameters including sex, age, and whether the patient is well or ill (and, if ill, whether it is a chronic or acute situation). Additionally, efficiency of absorption of a particular type of product and the quality of its individual ingredients are two major considerations for choosing appropriate specific agents for an individual's medical situation.

Anyone on prescription medication should first consult their physician prior to starting any new therapy, including nutraceuticals. Furthermore, anyone with malignancy should consult their physician or oncologist prior to beginning, or continuing, any hormone therapy program.

Finally, please be mindful that just because a product is natural doesn't mean it's safe for everyone. A small portion of the general population may react adversely to components in nutraceuticals (especially herbal products). A complete inventory of interventions utilized by a patient should be maintained by physicians and health practitioners dispensing anti-aging medical care.

JOIN the American Academy of Anti-Aging Medicine (A4M)

With 18,500 physician and scientist members from 85 nations worldwide, A4M is the world's leading medical society dedicated to the advancement of technology to detect, prevent, and treat aging related disease and to promote research into methods to retard and optimize the human aging process. Complete and return the Application for New Membership at the back of this book, or visit **www.worldhealth.net** to transact your membership via the Internet.

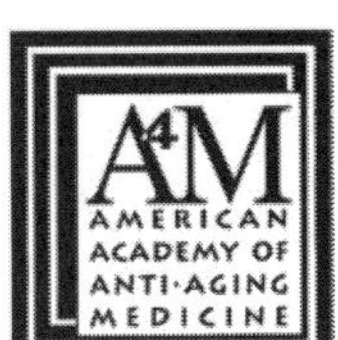

Established 1992

The Top Ten Natural Immune Enhancers

Natural immune enhancement via dietary supplements aims to strengthen an individual's overall immune function, reduce the viral load, and control inflammation. It also may boost antioxidant protection and optimize cellular processes.

As such, we consider the following as the Top Ten Natural Immune Enhancers to be:

- Arabinogalactan
- Epicor™
- Green tea
- Glutathione
- ImmunoMax
- Inositol hexaphosphate (IP6)
- Lactoferrin
- Mushrooms (Maitake, Shitake)
- Oregano oil
- Selenium

The "Immunity Desk Reference" provides concise monographs describing these natural supplements as well as more than 60 additional natural, non-toxic immune-enhancing strategies.

Hormones

DEHYDROEPIANDROSTERONE (DHEA)

DHEA is the most abundant steroid in the human body, and is involved in the manufacture of testosterone, estrogen, progesterone, and corticosterone. The decline of DHEA with age parallels that of HGH, so by age 65, your body makes only 10 to 20% of what it did at age 20. DHEA appears to be a potent immune system booster. Chiu *et al* found that it rejuvenated many measurements of immune function in mice, including the production of T-cells (white blood cells that are crucial to the immune system) white blood cell crucial to the immune system), interleukin-2 (a chemical messenger called a cytokine that can improve the body's natural response to disease), and other immune factors, which decline with age. Several studies have shown that DHEA treatment reverses the age-related defect in the immunity of old mice against influenza, however results in humans have been not as conclusive.

Human skin (and other tissues) contains enzymes that convert DHEA to 7-keto DHEA, which is almost identical in structure to DHEA. Research on 7-keto DHEA suggests that it may prove useful for immune enhancement/modulation, Alzheimer's disease, and weight loss. Results of a study by Lardy *et al* revealed that 7-keto DHEA increases interleukin-2 production, and is better at doing so than DHEA. Interleukin-2 is a very important player in the immune system as it activates the immune system to fight invading pathogens.

Dosing

Therapeutic Daily Amount: DHEA: Exact dosages have not been clearly established. Dosages commonly range between 25 to 150 mg, but it is best to start at the low-dose end of about 25 to 50 mg per day and raise the dosage later if needed. For best results, take in divided doses three or four times a day. It is important to have your DHEA levels measured every two to three months by your personal anti-aging physician. Some physicians also recommend that people taking DHEA should have their liver enzymes measured regularly.

7-keto DHEA: Most sources recommend taking 100 mg twice daily, however some physicians think that a lower dose, such as 25mg to 50mg daily with occasional breaks, may be more appropriate.

Side Effects/Contraindications: DHEA: Side effects caused by doses at the high end of the recommended daily intake (25-150 mg per day) include acne, increased facial hair, and increased perspiration. Less common side effects reported with DHEA supplementation include: breast tenderness, weight gain, mood alteration, headache, oily skin, and menstrual irregularities. Children, adolescents, pregnant and lactating women should not take DHEA. People with breast or prostate cancer, or a family history of these conditions, and those suffering from benign prostatic hyperplasia (BPH), other cancers, or endometriosis should also avoid supplementing with DHEA. The hormone can interfere with dihydrotestosterone and estrogen levels and large doses can cause liver damage.

7-keto DHEA: Davidson *et al* conducted a safety study of 7-keto DHEA in humans. Results showed that 7-keto DHEA was not associated with any negative effects at levels up to 200 mg per day for eight weeks. However, the long-term safety of 7-keto DHEA has not been demonstrated in humans. As 7-keto DHEA is chemically related to steroid hormones, the potential for adverse effects must be considered. Furthermore 7-keto DHEA is know to increase levels of thyroid hormone, and this could, theoretically, result in adverse effects on the heart or promote bone loss. For these reasons, people wishing to take 7-keto DHEA, particularly those who have a thyroid disorder or are taking thyroid hormone, should consult their physician. Pregnant women, nursing women, and people with cancer should not take 7-keto DHEA.

HUMAN GROWTH HORMONE (HGH)

Levels of HGH, which is secreted by the pituitary gland, decrease with age at the rate of about 14% per decade after age 30. In addition to assisting in DNA repair and rejuvenating the immune system, HGH replacement decreases fat tissue and increases lean tissue, increases bone density, promotes heart health, and improves mood. HGH benefits the immune system in several different ways. In 1985, Dr. Keith Kelley, showed that injections of cells that secrete HGH effectively renewed the shrivelled thymus gland (a small endocrine gland located in the upper chest that regulates the development of some immune system cells) in old rats so that it was as large and robust as that of young rats. HGH has been shown to: aid the manufacture of new antibodies (proteins produced by the immune system that recognize and help to fight infection), increase the production of T-cells (white blood cells that are crucial to the immune system) white blood cell crucial to the immune system) and interleukin-2 (a chemical messenger called a cytokine that can improve the body's natural response to disease), increase the proliferation and activity of disease-fighting white blood cells, increase the activity of anti-cancer natural killer cells (a type of white blood cell that destroys tumor cells and cells infected with certain organisms), stimulate bacteria-fighting macrophages (a type of white blood cell that protects the body against infection), and increase the maturation of neutrophils (a type of white blood cell that plays a central role in the defense of a host against infection by engulfing and killing foreign microorganisms.)

Dosing

Therapeutic Daily Amount: HGH is given via injection, because it would be inactivated by the stomach's hydrochloric acid if given by mouth. Therapeutic dose is determined by body weight, although the average weekly dose is approximately 4 IUs per week. Comparable, though less dramatic benefits may be achievable through HGH nutritionals (HGH secretagogues and amino acid precursors of HGH), and Human Growth Factors (hGf) that contain cytokinetic-promoting nutrients that promote youthful metabolism and cellular function and repair.

Side Effects/Contraindications: Side effects may include bloating, edema, carpal tunnel syndrome, gynecomastia (abnormal enlargement of breasts in men), slight decrease in response to insulin, slight increase in blood pressure, hypertension accompanied by headaches and swelling of the optic nerve and decrease in thyroid hormone production. All side effects seen in adults receiving HGH for Adult Growth Hormone Deficiency Syndrome (AGHD) were eliminated by the reduction or cessation of the use of HGH.

MELATONIN

Melatonin is secreted by the pineal gland, a small organ set behind and between the eyes. It affects many organs including the thymus, the pituitary, and the hypothalamus. Melatonin plays a major role in setting the body's internal clock and is vital for sleep. Melatonin is also important for the functioning of the immune system. Chen *et al* found that rats fed a diet supplemented with melatonin showed an increase in the production of interleukin-2 (a chemical messenger called a cytokine that can improve the body's natural response to disease), and thymocytes (cells that mature to become T-lymphocytes, which are responsible for attacking infectious invaders.) The results of this study also showed that melatonin suppresses an inflammatory response that causes arthritis in rats. Maestroni found that melatonin administered to lab animals enhances the release of Th1 cells (helper cells that coordinate the immune response to infectious agents). While in humans, Maestroni observed that melatonin enhances the production of interleukin-6 (a chemical messenger called a cytokine that activates B-lymphocytes, which secrete antibodies in response to infectious agents.) Taken together, these findings suggest that melatonin plays a role in mounting the proper immune defense when an organism is exposed to infectious agents.

Dosing

Therapeutic Daily Amount: Melatonin is widely available in drug-store chains in both capsules and slow-release preparations. Therapeutic doses range from 0.5-5mg per day. However, finding the right dose of melatonin is a matter of trial and error, thus use of this hormone is best conducted under the guidance of a qualified anti-aging physician.

Side Effects/Contraindications: Melatonin can exacerbate certain medical conditions, and some people who self-administer melatonin may suffer from lethargy or problems concentrating ("hangover" effect) the morning after taking it, suggesting that proper modulation of dosing to avoid discomfort is warranted. Taking doses that are far beyond physiologic or replacement doses may slow or inhibit your own natural production and release of the hormone. Melatonin causes sleepiness, so it should be taken only at bedtime. Women seeking to become pregnant, pregnant women, children, or people who are on prescription steroids, who have mental illness, depression, severe allergies, autoimmune diseases (such as multiple sclerosis), immune system cancers (such as lymphoma and leukemia), or any metastatic diseases that being are treated by medication should not take melatonin supplements. In 2002, Sutherland *et al* warned that melatonin might not be appropriate for people with nocturnal asthma. In this type of asthma, breathing is most difficult around 3 or 4 o'clock in the morning and causes an interruption in sleep. Tests on white blood cells from nocturnal asthmatics revealed that they released inflammation-triggering chemicals thought to be involved in airway constriction when exposed to melatonin.

THYMIC PROTEINS

Thymic proteins are produced by the thymus gland, which plays an important role in the immune system. The hormonal output of the thymus gland diminishes after the age of 25, thus impairing the immune system and increasing a person's susceptibility to tumors, rheumatic disease, and age-related disease. Thymic proteins have been shown to reverse thymic atrophy and restore levels of immunity to more youthful levels. Strengthening the immune system with thymic protein is believed to lead to increased ability to ward off infections from colds and flu to hepatitis and HIV. Thymic protein is thought to be particularly useful for the treatment of flu as it activates a type of white blood cells called T4-helper cells, which kill the flu virus in the early stages of replication

Dosing

Therapeutic Daily Amount: The standard dosage for healthy people is 2-4 micrograms per day. For prevention and treatment of influenza, a daily dose of 8-12 micrograms is recommended upon the first sign of symptoms.

Side Effects/Contraindications: Patients taking large doses of steroid hormones should avoid thymic proteins.

VITAMINS

VITAMIN A

Vitamin A is a fat-soluble vitamin that participates in numerous biological functions. Numerous studies point to the value of Vitamin A in boosting immunity. Research suggests that retinyl acetate, a form of vitamin A found naturally in food, primes the immune system. Coutsoudis *et al* studied the effect of vitamin A supplementation on selected factors of immunity in children measles, and results showed that children receiving the vitamin were significantly less likely to die and had markedly higher numbers of lymphocytes and Immunoglobulin G antibodies (proteins used by the immune system to identify and neutralize foreign objects like bacteria and viruses) to measles. Vitamin A has also been shown to enhance T-helper cell (a type of white blood cell that helps the body fight off certain infections) type 2 mediated immune responses, a finding that suggests that it may be useful in treating bacterial and parasitic infections, and mucosal infections. Vitamin A is found only in animal tissues; although its precursor beta-carotene (provitamin A) can be found in certain fruits and vegetables. Fish liver oils (as in cod liver oil), liver, milk, cream, cheese, butter, and eggs are good natural sources of vitamin A.

Dosing
Therapeutic Daily Amount: 7,000 - 10,000 I.U. The RDA is 3,000 IU (900mcg) for men, and 2,300 IU (700mcg) for women. The European RDA is 800mcg. People over the age of 65 and those with liver disease are advised to take no more than 15,000 IU of Vitamin-A. Vitamin A toxicity can be serious, thus, it is important to ensure that the recommended dose is not exceeded. Many nutritionally-based health professionals report success with short-term elevated doses of vitamin A in the range of up to 400,000 IUs for 4 to 5 days.
Side Effects/Contraindications: Women who are planning to become pregnant or those who are in the first three months of pregnancy should not eat liver, or take vitamin A supplements, unless told to do so by a physician, as too much vitamin A can cause birth defects. Results of a clinical trial by Cartmel *et al* showed that people taking 25,000 IU of vitamin A each day for approximately four years experienced an 11% increase in triglycerides, a 3% increase in total cholesterol and a 1% decrease in "good" HDL cholesterol, suggesting that people at high risk of developing heart disease should be cautious when thinking about taking supplementary vitamin-A. Melhus *et al* found that a daily intake of just 5,000 IU of vitamin-A (the US RDA) was associated with a significant reduction in bone mineral density. The decrease in bone mineral density was so great that it approximately doubled the risk of hip fracture. While Michaelsson *et al* found that men in their 40s and 50s who have the highest blood levels of vitamin A are 2.5-times more likely than men with lower levels to break their hip when they are older. Based on these findings, people at high risk of developing osteoporosis – in particular menopausal and postmenopausal women – may benefit from taking beta-carotene supplements instead of vitamin A. Vitamin A should not be taken by people using the acne medications isotretinoin, resorcinol, topical sulfur, and tazarotene.

B VITAMINS

The immune-boosting B vitamins include: folic acid, B2 (riboflavin), B5 (pantothenic acid), B6 (pyridoxine), and B12 (cobalamin or cyanocobalamin.)

Folic Acid (vitamin B9): Folic acid is needed for RNA and DNA synthesis, red blood cell production, and the metabolism of protein. It also increases the activity and production of antibodies and may reduce susceptibility to infection. Supplementary folic acid may help to strengthen the immune system in older people. Results of a study published in January 2006 revealed that folic acid improves age-related decreases in lymphocyte (white blood cell) function. Folic acid is found in deep-green leafy vegetables, liver, brewer's yeast, whole grains, bran, asparagus, lima beans, lentils, and orange juice.

Dosing

Therapeutic Daily Dose: 400-800mcg (micrograms) combined with B-complex vitamin. RDA for men and women is 400mcg; women who are planning or who may become pregnant, and those in the first trimester of pregnancy are advised to take 600mcg of folic acid every day. The RDA for nursing women is 500mcg. The maximum safe levels are 400mcg (long-term usage), 700mcg (short-term usage). The National Academy of Sciences recommends that the daily intake of folic acid in adults should not exceed 1,000 mcg.

Side Effects/Contraindications: Very high doses of folic acid may trigger seizures in people with epilepsy, thus epileptics should seek a doctor's advice before taking supplements.

Vitamin B2 (riboflavin): Vitamin B2 is manufactured in the body by the intestinal flora, although very small quantities are stored in the body. Vitamin B2 plays an important role in the metabolism of amino acids, fatty acids, and carbohydrates. There is evidence to suggest that it may play a role in red blood cell formation and antibody production. Vitamin B2 has been shown to enhance host resistance to bacterial infections in mice. Vitamin B2 is believed to benefit the immune system by stimulating the multiplication of neutrophils (a type of white blood cell that plays a central role in the defense of a host against infection by engulfing and killing foreign microorganisms) and monocytes (large, circulating, white blood cells that act as scavengers capable of destroying invading bacteria or other foreign material), and by activating macrophages (a type of white blood cell that protects the body against infection). Natural sources of riboflavin include brewer's yeast, almonds, organ meats, whole grains, wheat germ, wild rice, mushrooms, soybeans, milk, yogurt, eggs, broccoli, brussel sprouts, and spinach. Flour and cereals are often fortified with riboflavin.

Dosing

Therapeutic Daily Dose: The RDA is 1.3 mg for men, 1.1 mg for women, 1.4 mg for pregnant women, and 1.6 mg for women who are breastfeeding.

Side Effects/Contraindications: Riboflavin is not associated with any serious side effects. However, prolonged use of very high doses may cause itching, numbness, burning or prickling sensations, and sensitivity to light. Riboflavin should not be taken at the same time as the antibiotic tetracycline, anti-malarial medications such as chloroquine and mefloquine, the anti-cancer drug doxorubicin, the Parkinson's drug selegiline, and sulfa-containing medications, for example, trimethoprim-sulfamethoxazole.

Vitamin B5 (pantothenic acid): Like the other water-soluble B vitamins, B5 plays an important role in the breakdown of fats and carbohydrates for energy. Vitamin B5 is also vital to the manufacture of red blood cells, antibodies, and the stress-related hormones produced in the adrenal glands. It is sometimes referred to as the "anti-stress" vitamin because it is believed to enhance the activity of the immune system and increase the body's ability to withstand stressful conditions. The biologically active form of pantothenic acid is pantethine, which can be purchased as a supplement in tablet form. The best food sources of vitamin B5 are brewer's yeast, corn, cauliflower, kale, broccoli, tomatoes, avocado, legumes, lentils, egg yolks, beef, turkey, duck, chicken, milk, split peas, peanuts, soybeans, sweet potatoes, sunflower seeds, whole-grain breads and cereals, lobster, wheat germ, and salmon.

Dosing
Therapeutic Daily Dose: The RDA is 5 mg. However, 250 mg twice daily is recommended for adrenal support during times of stress and illness.
Side Effects/Contraindications: No serious side effects are associated with vitamin B5. Vitamin B5 should not be taken at the same time as the antibiotic drug tetracycline.

Vitamin B6 (pyridoxine): Vitamin B6 metabolizes proteins, fats, and carbohydrates, and is essential for maintaining a healthy nervous system. It is also required for the formation of hemoglobin in red blood cells and antibodies that help fight infection. Like vitamin B5, vitamin B6 is considered an "anti-stress" vitamin because it is believed to enhance the activity of the immune system and increase the body's ability to withstand stressful conditions. Vitamin B6 is found in brewer's yeast, sunflower seeds, wheat germ, liver and other organ meats, blackstrap molasses, bananas, walnuts, roasted peanuts, lentils, soybeans, avocados, carrots, brown rice, bran, canned tuna and salmon. Breakfast cereals are often fortified with vitamin B6. US government surveys suggest that as many as one-third of US adults suffer from vitamin B6 deficiency.

Dosing

Therapeutic Daily Dose: 50-100mg combined with a B-complex supplement. The RDA for men and women aged 19 to 50 years is 1.3 mg. For men aged 51 years and older the RDA is 1.7 mg, and for women aged 51 years and older it is 1.5 mg. Doses of up to 100mg per day on a long-term basis are safe, although no adverse effects have been seen with doses of up to 200mg. Doses in excess of 200mg may cause neurologic disorders.

Side Effects/Contraindications: No side effects are associated with recommended dosages of vitamin B6. Vitamin B6 can cause neurological disorders, such as loss of sensation in legs and imbalance, when taken in doses of 200 mg or more per day over a long period of time. However, discontinuing the use of such high doses usually leads to a complete recovery within 6 months. There have also been reports of allergic skin reactions to high doses of vitamin B6 supplements, however such reactions are extremely rare. Vitamin B6 should not be used in conjunction with the antibiotic tetracycline, levodopa (a medication used to treat Parkinson's disease), phenytoin (a medication used to treat seizures), and hydralazine (a medication used to treat high blood pressure.)

Vitamin B12 (cobalamin or cyanocobalamin): Vitamin B12 is required for the production of red and white blood cells and blood platelets (thrombocytes), the manufacture of substances needed for correct cell functioning, and the metabolism of nutrients necessary for cell growth. It is essential for the recycling of certain enzymes that maintain the health of blood, nerve, and other cells. It also aids the metabolism of proteins, fats, and carbohydrates. Like vitamin B5 and vitamin B6, vitamin B12 is considered an "anti-stress" vitamin because it is believed to enhance the activity of the immune system and increase the body's ability to withstand stressful conditions. Vitamin B12 is found in organ meats, liver, beef, pork, eggs, whole milk, cheese, whole wheat bread, and fish. As vitamin B12 is not found in plant foods unless they are fortified (e.g. breakfast cereal), vegans are likely to benefit from vitamin B12 supplementation.

Dosing

Therapeutic Daily Dose: 500-1,000 mcg (micrograms) with a complete B-complex vitamin. Sublingual form is best absorbed with tablets placed under the tongue. RDA is 2.4 mcg. For pregnant women the RDA is 2.6mcg, while for lactating women it is 2.8mcg. The European RDA is 1 mcg. The National Academy of Science of the US recommends that adults over age 50 meet most of their recommended intake with synthetic B12 from fortified foods or vitamin supplements. 3,000 mcg (long and short term -- no adverse effect established) is the generally accepted upper safe limit, although no official tolerable upper intake level has been established.

Side Effects/Contraindications: Oral vitamin B12 is not associated with any side effects. However, serious allergic reactions to injections of vitamin B12 have been reported, although such side effects are rare. Patients with the rare eye disease Lebers disease should consult their doctor before taking vitamin B12. Vitamin B12 should not be taken at the same time as the antibiotic tetracycline

VITAMIN C (ASCORBIC ACID)

Vitamin C is a potent antioxidant and protects against free radical cellular damage. Thanks to Linus Pauling's work on vitamin C and the common cold, vitamin C is probably the best known of the immune-boosting nutrients.   Vitamin C (1,000–6,000 mg/day) is purported to shorten the duration of colds and flu, and help fight secondary bacterial infections that can accompany a cold. Research by Braun *et al* revealed that 67% of those surveyed believed that taking supplementary vitamin C helped to reduce cold symptoms. Vitamin C may also reduce the symptoms and duration of infection of other viruses such as mumps, herpes, measles and the flu. Vitamin C is found in rose hips, citrus fruit and juices, strawberries, blueberries, cantaloupes, tomatoes, and raw vegetables such as red bell peppers.

Dosing
Therapeutic Daily Dose: 1,000-2,000mg depending on your need. RDA is 90mg for men and 75mg for women. For the treatment of influenza, a daily dose of 1,000–6,000 mg is recommended. Research suggests that blood levels of vitamin do not increase further when vitamin C doses exceed 250-500 mg per day. Vitamin C may enhance the effects of some chemotherapy drugs, however cancer patients should always consult their oncologist before taking dietary supplements.
Side Effects/Contraindications: No side effects are associated with vitamin C, however large doses of the vitamin can deplete the body's supplies of the essential nutrient copper. People with a glucose-6-phosphate dehydrogenase deficiency, iron overload (hemosiderosis or hemochromatosis), history of kidney stones, or kidney failure should consult their doctor before taking supplementary vitamin C. High doses of vitamin C can cause kidney stones in people with a history of the condition and those who regularly undergo hemodialysis. Women taking the contraceptive pill should not take excessively large doses of vitamin C as it may reduce the effectiveness of the pill. People taking ampicillin, indomethacin, salsalate (a drug used to manage arthritis), warfarin, or tetracycline should not take supplementary vitamin C without consulting their doctor, this is because vitamin C may increase or decrease the effectiveness of these drugs.

VITAMIN D (ERGOCALCIFEROL)

Vitamin D is a fat-soluble vitamin that enhances the absorption of calcium from the intestine and the utilization of calcium and phosphorus in the body, thus, ensuring that calcium and phosphorus levels are high enough to support the constant breakdown and rebuilding of bone tissue. It is therefore essential for strong and healthy bones. Vitamin D is a potent immune system modulator. Research has shown that the vitamin D receptor is expressed by most cells of the immune system, including T-cells (white blood cells that are crucial to the immune system) white blood cell crucial to the immune system) and antigen-presenting cells (cells that present foreign substances capable of eliciting an immune response, such as bacteria, to the immune system), such as dendritic cells (specialized cells that present antigens (foreign substances) to specific cells of the immune system) and macrophages (a type of white blood cell that protects the body against infection.) There is also evidence to suggest that vitamin D exerts a variety of effects on immune system function that may enhance innate immunity and help to prevent the development of autoimmunity.

Vitamin D3 (cholecalciferol) is the natural form of vitamin D, which is manufactured by the body when 7-dehydrocholesterol present in the skin reacts with ultraviolet light (specifically UVB). Under the right conditions, the body can manufacture as much as 20,000 IU of vitamin D3 within a matter of minutes. However, merely being exposed to sunlight is not sufficient as only the UVB radiation in sunlight triggers vitamin D production, and UVB only reaches ground level in significant quantities when the sun is high in the sky. Therefore optimal conditions for vitamin D manufacture occur for only a few hours each day, and at higher latitudes, the sun is only high enough in the sky in summer. Therefore vitamin D levels plummet during the fall and winter in people living in temperate climates, such as North America and Europe. Some experts believe that exposing the body to sunlight and therefore ensuring that the body has a plentiful supply of vitamin D3 can reduce the risk of many cancers by more than 50%, and even help to reverse certain types of cancers. Vitamin D has also been linked with infectious diseases, such as influenza, as statistics show that epidemics tend to occur during the fall and winter – the same time at which vitamin D levels plummet. Two animal studies support the theory that vitamin D prevents the flu, however one animal study and one human study found no evidence to support the theory. Vitamin D is derived from sunshine (manufactured through the skin), cod liver oil, liver, and egg yolks. Margarine and cereals are often fortified with vitamin D.

Dosing

Therapeutic Daily Dose: 400-800 IU from cod liver oil. The RDA for vitamin D is 5 mcg (200 IU) a day for men and women aged 19 to 50, 10 mcg (400 IU) for those aged 51 to 70, and 15 mcg (600 IU) for people aged 71 and over. Hollis believes that the current RDA's for vitamin D are very inadequate when one considers that a 10-15 min whole-body exposure to peak summer sun will generate and release up to 20,000 IU vitamin D into the circulation. Hollis argues that did not evolve to live in a "sun-shy" culture, and therefore "normal" with respect to circulating vitamin D levels should not be defined by the current average or median population level. Hollis suggests that the requirements for vitamin D should be re-examined, and that reexamination may likely reveal the need for vitamin D intakes exceeding 2000 IU/d for adults. However, at present, the maximum daily intake of vitamin D is 10 mcg (long-term) and 50 mcg (short-term). A daily intake (both from fortified food and supplements) of more than 25 mcg (1,000 IU) of vitamin D is not currently advisable. Long-term consumption of vitamin D at doses greater than 25 mcg may cause high blood pressure, premature hardening of the arteries, bone pain, deterioration of bone, calcium build-up in muscles and soft tissues, kidney damage, excessive thirst, metal taste, poor appetite, weight loss, tiredness, sore eyes, itching skin, vomiting, diarrhea or constipation, a need to urinate, and muscle problems.

Side Effects/Contraindications: Pregnant or breast-feeding women should limit their vitamin D intake to no more than 20 mcg (800 IU) a day as higher doses have been linked to birth abnormalities. People taking antacids containing magnesium and thiazide diuretics, such as hydrochlorothiazide, should not use supplements. People with high blood calcium or phosphorus levels, heart problems, and kidney disease, such consult their physician before taking supplementary vitamin D.

VITAMIN E

Vitamin E is a fat-soluble vitamin known for its potent antioxidant activity and for its positive effects on heart health, immune cells, and resistance to infection. Research suggests that vitamin E may boost the immune system, and increase the immune response in older people. Vitamin E is found in wheat germ oil, soybean oil, safflower oil, peanuts, whole grains (wheat, rice, oats), green, leafy vegetables, cabbage, spinach, asparagus, broccoli, and egg yolks.

Dosing

Therapeutic Daily Dose: 400-1,200 IU. To obtain these potencies, one should use natural vitamin E supplements providing a blend of alpha, gamma (found to have the highest antioxidant free-radical scavenging activity), beta, and delta tocopherols. The US RDA for vitamin E has recently been updated and is now 15 mg (22.5 IU) for both men and women. The maximum daily dose is 800 IU (long and short-term). The daily tolerable upper intake level for adults established by the National Academy of Sciences is 1,000 mg of vitamin E, which is equivalent to 1,500 IU of natural vitamin E or 1,100 IU of synthetic vitamin E.

Side Effects/Contraindications: Vitamin E should not be taken in combination with anticoagulant (blood-thinning) drugs such as warfarin and aspirin. People taking tricyclic antidepressants, the antipsychotic medication chlorpromazine, beta-blockers, and anti-malarial medication should consult their physician before taking supplementary vitamin E. Due to vitamin E's blood-thinning properties people scheduled for elective surgery (including dental surgery) are advised to avoid supplementary vitamin E for two days before and after surgery. Much controversy concerning the safety of vitamin E supplementation arose following the publication of a study by Miller *et al* in 2005, in which supplementary vitamin E was linked to an increased risk of death in elderly people. It should be noted that the study population in Millers study was elderly and many of the participants had pre-existing serious illnesses, such as heart disease. Following the publication of the study by Miller *et al*, Hathcock *et al* published a review of the safety of both vitamin C and Vitamin E, in which the authors concluded: "The fact that adverse effects are rarely reported for vitamins E at amounts higher than the RDA is testimony to the safety of such dietary supplementation up to the upper limit. Several literature reviews have concluded, on the basis of a survey of published evidence, that such intake does not cause adverse side effects or create other safety issues...The recommendations are entirely based on the available scientific evidence; the main caveat is that healthy persons should not "routinely" take vitamin E in amounts higher than the upper limit. Beyond that, the recommendations support the consensus of published studies that vitamin E doses up to 1000 mg/day are safe for use by the general population."

MINERALS

MAGNESIUM

Magnesium is involved in hundreds of enzyme reactions, and a deficiency of this mineral can adversely affect the immune system. Magnesium participates in immune responses in numerous ways, for example the ability of immune cells to adhere to other substances, and the synthesis of immunoglobulins (proteins that act as antibodies) is dependent upon magnesium. Rich sources of magnesium include tofu, legumes, whole grains, green leafy vegetables, wheat bran, Brazil nuts, soybean flour, almonds, cashew nuts, blackstrap molasses, pumpkin and squash seeds, pine nuts, and black walnuts. Other good dietary sources of magnesium include peanuts, wholewheat flour, oat flour, beet greens, spinach, pistachio nuts, shredded wheat, bran cereals, oatmeal, bananas, baked potatoes (with skin), chocolate, and cocoa powder.

Dosing

Therapeutic Daily Dose: Magnesium supplementation is important for people taking diuretics and digitalis. Heavy drinkers and those concerned about osteoporosis may also benefit from taking supplements of the mineral. Many doctors recommend taking a supplement containing 250–350 mg each day. The RDA of magnesium is 400 mg a day for men aged 19 to 30, 420mg a day for men aged 31 to 70. For women, the RDA is 310 mg a day for those aged 19 to 30, and 320 mg for those aged 31 to 70. The European RDA is 300 mg. The upper limit is 350 mg – this is for magnesium obtained from supplementation only and not through the diet.

Side Effects/Contraindications: The most common problem caused by magnesium is diarrhea, however, the amounts of magnesium found in nutritional supplements are unlikely to cause such problems. Even so, it is recommended to take small doses of magnesium throughout the day to avoid diarrhea. It is extremely rare to overdose on magnesium from food alone. However, ingesting too much magnesium can cause serious health problems including nausea, vomiting, severely lowered blood pressure, slowed heart rate, deficiencies of other minerals, confusion, coma, and even death. People with kidney disease or heart disease, and those taking antibiotics or drugs used to treat osteoporosis should consult their doctor before taking supplementary magnesium.

SELENIUM – A Top Ten Natural Immune Enhancer

Selenium is an essential trace element, necessary for growth and protein synthesis. It helps to increase the effectiveness of vitamin E, and acts as an antioxidant to protect cells from the free radical damage that causes aging and is linked to many age-related diseases. Research suggests that selenium is vital for the proper functioning of the immune system, and that it can increase levels of white blood cells, therefore enhancing the body's ability to fight illness and infection. Selenium may also inhibit viral replication. A number of studies have found that selenium deficiency is linked to increased occurrence or progression of viral infections, thus supporting the theory that the mineral inhibits viral replication. Broome *et al* found that selenium supplementation improved immune function and increased the rate of clearance of poliovirus vaccine in humans. A study of elderly men and women by Girodon revealed that those who received zinc and selenium supplements demonstrated a better immune response to the influenza vaccine than those who received placebo. Thus suggesting that supplementary selenium and zinc may help to boost immunity in older people and improve their resistance to infections, such as influenza. Good dietary sources of selenium include: Brewer's yeast and wheat germ, liver, butter, fish (mackeral, tuna, halibut, flounder, herring, smelts) and shellfish (oysters, scallops and lobster), garlic, whole grains, sunflower seeds, and Brazil nuts.

Dosing

Therapeutic Daily Dose: The RDA of selenium is 55 mcg for women and 70 mcg for men, however many experts recommend a daily intake of 100-200mcg. The maximum safe level is 200mcg for long-term usage and 700mcg for short-term usage. Supplementation at levels greater than 800 mcg a day may be toxic. The Food and Nutrition Board states that overt selenium toxicity may occur in humans ingesting 2,400-3,000mcg.

Side Effects/Contraindications: Side effects are rare, but can include dizziness, nausea, brittle fingernails, and hair loss. People taking cholesterol-lowering medications, such as statins, should consult their physician before taking supplementary selenium as it may reduce their effectiveness.

ZINC

Zinc is one of the most important trace elements in the body as it plays a role in many biological functions. Zinc promotes resistance to infections, particularly in aging, a time when the immune system slows down. Zinc has been shown to increase the activity of natural killer cells (a type of white blood cell that destroys tumor cells and cells infected with certain organisms) and to boost the production of antibodies (proteins produced by the immune system that recognize and help to fight infection) in response to infection. Research suggests that it can help immune cells to fight a cold, and may relieve cold symptoms when taken as a supplement. Research by Mossad revealed that a zinc-based nasal spray was able to cut the duration of a cold in half if treatment was started within two days of the onset of symptoms.

Dosing

Therapeutic Daily Dose: 15-50 mg (take with copper to yield a zinc to copper ratio of 10:1). The RDA is 11 mg for men and 8 mg for women. Coffee drinkers should take zinc supplements at least one hour before or two hours after drinking coffee, as it reduces the body's ability to absorb zinc by 50%. The maximum safe level for long-term use is 15 mg, for short-term use, 50 mg can be taken safely, although doses of 50 mg and more should only be taken under medical advice and supervision. Supplementation at levels greater than 150 mg/day may suppress immunity and cause other side effects.

Side Effects/Contraindications: High doses of zinc affect the absorption of iron and copper, suppress the immune system, raise LDL cholesterol (the "bad" form of cholesterol), and lower HDL cholesterol (the "good" form of cholesterol) levels. Zinc should be taken with food to avoid irritating the stomach. People with liver damage or an intestinal disorder should consult their doctor before taking supplementary zinc. Zinc should not be taken with corticosteroids, cyclosporine, or other medications intended to suppress the immune system.

Zinc may reduce the effectiveness of NSAIDs (nonsteroidal anti-inflammatory drugs, for example aspirin and ibuprofen) therefore people taking such drugs should consult their physician before taking supplementary zinc. Results of several studies conducted over the last few years have linked zinc to Alzheimer's disease. However, one study found that the zinc appeared to improve mental performance in Alzheimer's patients. Until the effect of zinc on Alzheimer's is understood more clearly, people diagnosed with Alzheimer's and those deemed at high risk of developing the disease may wish to avoid taking supplementary zinc.

AMINO ACIDS

ARGININE

Arginine is a non-essential amino acid that the body can synthesize in the liver, however in times of stress or trauma arginine becomes an essential amino acid. The end-products of arginine metabolism produced by the enzymes arginase, arginine decarboxylase (ADC), and nitric oxide synthase (NOS) have been shown to play roles in wound healing, immune response, tumor biology, and the regulation of inflammation. Arginine boosts the immune system, and therefore is useful for people recovering from illness or surgery. Arginine is a well-known T lymphocyte (a type of white blood cell crucial to the immune system) stimulator. Daly *et al* found that supplemental arginine significantly enhanced the mean post-surgery T-lymphocyte response and increased the mean CD4 phenotype (an important type of white blood cell that recognizes antigens (foreign substances) on the surface of virus-infected cells) in surgical patients. Li *et al* observed that supplementation of surgical patients with arginine around the time of surgery was able to enhance immune function by increasing interleukin-2 (a chemical messenger called a cytokine that can improve the body's natural response to disease) production. Results of a study by Barbul *et al*, where healthy volunteers were given 30 grams of arginine each day led the authors to conclude: "Supplemental dietary arginine is a safe nutritional stimulator of lymphocyte (white blood cell) immune reactivity in healthy human beings."

Dosing
Therapeutic Daily Dose: A typical therapeutic dosage of arginine is 2-3 g per day. Oral supplementation with L-arginine at daily doses of up to 15 grams is generally well tolerated. Most people do not need to take supplementary arginine. People suffering from serious burns, infections, or other trauma may need extra arginine, however a doctor should decide the dosage. Doses used in the studies above to improve immune function ranged between 25 and 43 grams per day.
Side Effects/Contraindications: The most common adverse reactions of higher doses — from 15 to 30 grams daily — are nausea, abdominal cramps and diarrhea. Individuals with renal or hepatic insufficiency and those with insulin-dependent diabetes should avoid large doses of arginine. As should people who are allergic to eggs, milk, or wheat. Some doctors

suggest that people with herpes should not take arginine supplements, because it aids herpes virus replication. Arginine should not be taken in combination with lysine, as lysine is an antagonist of arginine. Arginine can interfere with the metabolism of lysine, which can reactivate the herpes simplex virus. People taking non-steroidal anti-inflammatory drugs (NSAID's) such as aspirin, and drugs that alter potassium levels, for example ACE inhibitors, should be cautious if taking supplementary arginine. People with kidney or liver disease should consult their doctor before taking supplementary arginine.

CYSTEINE (N-ACETYL CYSTEINE [NAC])

Cysteine is a non-essential amino acid that can be manufactured in the liver. Cysteine may boost the immune system, promote the metabolism of fats and production of muscle tissue, aid healing after surgery, promote hair growth, and prevent hair loss. N-acetyl cysteine (NAC) is a modified form of cysteine. NAC's power as an immune system booster stems from its ability to enhance the production of the enzyme glutathione, a potent antioxidant vital for the correct functioning of the immune system. NAC may also reduce the severity and duration of influenza by thinning mucus and weakening the flu virus. De Flora et al gave 262 people 600 mg NAC or placebo twice daily for six months. Results showed that treatment with NAC resulted in a significant decrease in the frequency of influenza-like episodes, severity, and length of time confined to bed. The results led the authors to conclude: "Administration of N-acetylcysteine during the winter, thus, appears to provide a significant attenuation of influenza and influenza-like episodes, especially in elderly high-risk individuals." Cysteine is obtained in the diet from beans, brewer's yeast, broccoli, Brussels sprouts, dairy products, eggs, fish, garlic, legumes, meat, nuts, onions, red peppers, seafood, seeds, soy, whey, and whole grains.

Dosing

Therapeutic Daily Dose: Optimal levels of NAC and cysteine have not been determined. 250 to 1,500 mg of NAC per day has been used in clinical studies with no adverse effects. A maximum safe level has not been established, however there are no known signs of toxicity from cysteine. NAC appears to be a very safe supplement even in high doses, however an animal study found that 60-100 times the normal dose could cause liver injury. Note: NAC is known to have antioxidant activity, however one study found that daily doses of 1.2g or more increased oxidative stress. For the treatment of influenza a dose of 500 mg thrice daily is recommended.

Side Effects/Contraindications: People with diabetes mellitus and allergies to eggs, milk, or wheat should not take supplementary cysteine. People taking the drug may experience severe headaches when taking NAC. Cysteine supplements must be taken with vitamin C to prevent cysteine being converted to cystine, which may form kidney or bladder stones. People with kidney or liver disease should consult their doctor before taking supplementary cysteine.

GLUTAMINE

The most abundant amino acid in muscles and blood, glutamine provides fuel for various cells of the immune system and is a critical component in wound repair. The body can make glutamine, but may not make enough when the body is under stress. Preliminary evidence suggests that glutamine might help prevent infections in people who are over-stressed and athletes who are overtrained – and thus immunosuppressed. Research has shown that glutamine enhances lymphocyte (white blood cell) function. Results of a study of gastric cancer patients by Chen *et al* revealed that 7 days of treatment with an immunonutrition formula enriched with glutamine, arginine (an amino acid), and omega-3 fatty acids led to increased levels of immunoglobulins (proteins that act as antibodies), CD4 cells (an important type of white blood cell that recognizes antigens (foreign substances) on the surface of virus-infected cells), and interleukin-2 (a chemical messenger called a cytokine that can improve the body's natural response to disease), and lower levels of interleukin-6 (a pro-inflammatory chemical messenger) and tumor necrosis factor (TNF-alpha – a pro-inflammatory chemical messenger that kills tumor cells). Griffiths *et al* found that intravenous glutamine supplementation increased the survival rate of critically ill people. There is also evidence that supplemental glutamine can help to maintain immune system function in critically ill patients. Thus, glutamine may be useful as a nutritional supplement for people undergoing recovery from illness. Glutamine has also been shown to increase levels of the enzyme glutathione, a potent antioxidant vital for the correct functioning of the immune system. Glutamine is found naturally in beans, brewer's yeast, brown rice, dairy products, eggs, fish, legumes, meat, nuts, seafood, seeds, soy, whey, and whole grains.

Dosing
Therapeutic Daily Dose: Doses range from 1.5 to 6g daily, divided into several separate doses. The majority of healthy people do not need to take supplementary glutamine. A maximum safe level has not been established, however glutamine is generally regarded as safe.
Side Effects/Contraindications: People who are hypersensitive to monosodium glutamate (MSG) should use glutamine with caution, as the body metabolises glutamine into glutamate. Individuals taking antiseizure medications, for example carbamazepine, phenobarbital, Dilantin (phenytoin), Mysoline (primidone), and valproic acid (Depakene),

should only take supplementary glutamine under medical supervision. People with kidney or liver disease should consult their doctor before taking supplementary glutamine.

GLUTATHIONE — A Top Ten Natural Immune Enhancer

Glutathione is a tripeptide composed of the three amino acids glycine, glutamic acid (glutamate), and cysteine. Glutathione has been called the "master antioxidant." In addition to its own potent antioxidant powers glutathione helps to recycle other antioxidants such as vitamins C and E. Thus, glutathione can help to protect against aging, cancer, and other diseases caused by oxidative damage. Glutathione plays an important role in the regulation of immune cells, and results of several studies suggest that glutathione has antiviral properties. Research has shown that glutathione inhibits activation and replication of the influenza virus. Scientists from Emory University reported at the Experimental Biology 2000 meeting in San Diego that glutathione, could help prevent infection by the influenza virus if administered directly to the tissues lining the mouth and upper airway. The scientists suggested that glutathione concentrated in a lozenge or spray might be the most effective way to use the compound as a flu preventive. It has also been shown to inhibit activation of the HIV virus and the herpes simplex virus-1 (HSV-1).

Dosing

Therapeutic Daily Dose: People with a proven glutathione deficiency should be treated by a doctor, and may require intravenous or intramuscular injections. A maximum safe level for glutathione has not been established. Some research suggests that taking oral glutathione may not be the best way of raising blood glutathione levels. One study showed that healthy people could raise their blood glutathione levels by nearly 50% by taking 500mg of vitamin C each day for 2-weeks. Other nutritional compounds that may help to boost glutathione levels include: alpha lipoic acid, glutamine, methionine, S-adenosyl methionine (SAMe), and whey protein.

Side Effects/Contraindications: People with kidney or liver disease should consult their doctor before taking supplementary glutathione.

LYSINE

Lysine is an essential amino acid that is important for growth and bone development. It also promotes calcium absorption, maintains nitrogen balance, aids in the production of hormones, and collagen, and helps to build muscle tissue. Lysine is needed for the production of antibodies, and studies have shown that lysine-deficiency in animals is associated with a reduced antibody response and cell-mediated immune response to infection Lysine is a natural protease inhibitor (a compound that interferes with the ability of certain enzymes to break down proteins), and therefore it can help to prevent bacteria and viruses from replicating, and therefore limit infection. Several studies have found that regular use of lysine supplements may reduce the frequency and intensity of herpes virus flare-ups, and speed up the healing of sores, thus suggesting that the amino acid also has some antiviral properties. Beans, brewer's yeast, cheese, dairy products, eggs, fish, legumes, lima beans, meat, milk, nuts, potatoes, seafood, seeds, soy, whey, whole grains, and yeast, are natural sources of lysine.

Dosing

Therapeutic Daily Dose: Most people do not require lysine supplementation. For the treatment or prevention of influenza, some sources recommend a dose of 6000 mg each day – to be taken in three doses of 2000 mg at mealtimes. 1,000-3,000 mg of lysine per day is recommended for the treatment of herpes. A maximum safe dose has not been established. Lysine supplements should not be taken for any longer than 6 months, as prolonged use may cause an imbalance of the amino acid arginine.

Side Effects/Contraindications: People who are allergic to eggs, milk, or wheat, and diabetics should not take supplementary lysine. People with kidney disease or liver disease should consult their doctor before taking lysine.

PROLINE

Proline is a non-essential amino acid. Proline is a major constituent of collagen, and is therefore integral in the production and maintenance of collagen. Therefore, proline is necessary for maintaining the integrity of skin health and texture. Proline also aids in the healing and maintenance of cartilage, and the strengthening of tendons, joints, and muscles. Proline is thought to help regulate the immune system, and may also have antiviral properties. The best dietary sources of proline are dairy products.

Dosing

Therapeutic Daily Dose: Because proline is a non-essential amino acid, a RDA has not been established. Doses range between 0.5 and 2 grams. A maximum safe level has not been established.

Side Effects/Contraindications: There are no known side effects associated with proline. Excessive and prolonged intake of proline has not proven harmful in humans and little information exists concerning an acute overdose of proline. Pregnant and nursing women and people who suffer from the enzyme deficiency proline oxidase deficiency or Hyperprolinemia Type I (HP-I) should not take supplementary proline.

TAURINE

Taurine is a conditionally-essential nutrient. As such, taurine is derived directly from the breakdown of food but the body can produce its own stores from other pre-proteins (the amino acids methionine and cysteine) as well. Taurine boosts the immune system by stimulating the release of interleukin-1 (a chemical messenger called a cytokine that stimulates immune system cells that fight disease) in macrophages (a type of white blood cell that protects the body against infection), and increasing the phagocytic (ability to ingest and destroy foreign matter, including bacteria) and bactericidal (ability to destroy bacteria) activity of neutrophils (a type of white blood cell that plays a central role in the defense of a host against infection by engulfing and killing foreign microorganisms.). It also helps to detoxify toxic substances such as retinoids and environmental toxins. Brewer's yeast, dairy products, eggs, fish, meat, ox bile, and seafood, are natural sources of taurine.

Dosing
Therapeutic Daily Dose: The therapeutic dose ranges between 1.5-6 g a day. A maximum safe level has not been established.
Side Effects/Contraindications: Although rare, taurine can cause memory loss and depression of the central nervous system (CNS). People with kidney disease or liver disease should consult their doctor before taking taurine.

FATTY ACIDS

OMEGA-3 FATTY ACIDS (DHA & EPA)

Omega-3 fatty acids, which are found in primarily in fish oils but are also present in vegetable oils, are essential fatty acids. Therefore they are not made by the body and must be supplied by the diet or supplements. Omega-3 fatty acids have profound anti-inflammatory effects when taken at a therapeutic dosage. Omega-3's help curb an overactive immune system and thus are helpful in the treatment of autoimmune diseases such as rheumatoid arthritis, chronic inflammatory bowel disease, Crohn's disease, and psoriasis. Omega-3's are also effective in curbing the inflammatory response to severe burns, sepsis, systemic inflammatory response syndrome (SIRS) and asthma. Nordvik *et al* found that omega-3's can improve the clinical outcome for newly diagnosed multiple sclerosis patients. Omega-3's may confer greater resistance to common illnesses such as influenza and the common cold. Mackerel, salmon, sea bass, trout, herring, sardines, sablefish (black cod), anchovies, and tuna, as well as cod liver oil supplements, are rich sources of both DHA (docosahexaenoic acid) and EPA (eicosapentaenoic acid).

Dosing

Therapeutic Daily Dose: Eat oily fish several times a week for naturally occurring omega-3s and the nutrients that accompany them. Use canola oil in cooking and salad dressings. The majority of research into the effects of DHA and EPA in humans have used doses of at least 3g of DHA plus EPA supplements. To obtain a similar amount of DHA and EPA from fish oil it may be necessary to consume as much as 10g, as most fish oils contains only 18% EPA and 12% DHA. It is important to buy a good quality, mercury-free, fish oil supplement. A maximum safe dose has not established. Burns *et al* found that the maximum amount of fish oil tolerated by people being treated for cancer-related weight loss was roughly 21g per day. However, the maximum tolerated amount in people without cancer may well be different. High doses of fish oil (3 g and above) should only be taken if directed to do so by an expert.

Side Effects/Contraindications: Omega-3 fatty acids should be used cautiously by people who have a bleeding disorder, or take blood-thinning medications, as excessive amounts of omega-3 fatty acids may lead to bleeding. People who consume more than three grams of omega-3 fatty acids per day (equivalent to 3 servings of fish per day) may be at an increased risk for hemorrhagic stroke.

ALKYLGLYCEROLS

Alkylglycerols (AKG's) are lipids that stimulate the production of white blood cells and encourage the growth of antibodies. Alkylglycerols are considered critical to the development of a healthy immune system in children. Animal studies suggest that AKGs may inhibit cancer growth by selectively destroying cancer cells via their ability to induce apoptosis (cell suicide). Because of the immune system enhancing effects of alkylglycerols, they also help the body to fight bacterial, viral, and parasitic infections. AKGs are found in human breast milk, cow's milk, and the livers of most animals and fish. Shark liver contains an exceptionally high level of AKGs.

Dosing

Therapeutic Daily Dose: 500-1500mg per day
Side Effects/Contraindications: No side effects have been side with doses as high as 6000mg per day.

BOTANICAL AGENTS

ALOE

The Aloe Vera plant is native to North Africa. Aloes have been used all over the world throughout the ages for their various medicinal properties. Aloe is a biological response modifier (BRM), which means that it augments the immune response .The gel of the aloe leaf contains several chemicals, a polysaccharide, enzymes, nutrients, and other compounds that appear to fight bacteria and fungi, reduce inflammation, and encourage wound healing. Aloeride and acemannan, two isolated compounds in the gel of the aloe leaf, have been shown to stimulate the immune system and reduce the time it takes for skin to heal. Manufacturers sell the transparent gel from the plant's leaf as a topical remedy; they also process it into "juice" and pills, which are taken internally for gastrointestinal benefits or as a tonic.

Dosing

Therapeutic Daily Dose: Check product labels for dosage recommendations. Aloe juice products for oral consumption are generally considered safe, although drinking more than a pint a day may lead to diarrhea.

Side Effects/Contraindications: Gel preparations used topically have not been associated with side effects. Products made from the plant's latex can cause side effects such as intestinal cramping due to their laxative effect. Because of these side effects, the latex form of aloe should not be used by elderly people, children, pregnant or breastfeeding women, and anyone with inflammatory intestinal diseases, such as Crohn's disease, ulcerative colitis, or appendicitis.

ARABINOGALACTAN – A Top Ten Natural Immune Enhancer

Arabinogalactan (AG) is a phytochemical extracted from the timber of the larch tree. AG has a beneficial effect upon the immune system as it increases the activity of natural killer cells (a type of white blood cell that destroys tumor cells and cells infected with certain organisms), and other immune system components, thus helping the body to fight infection. AG also acts as a food supply for "friendly" bacteria, in that it helps to increase levels of "good" bacteria such as bifidobacteria and lactobacillus, while eliminating "bad" bacteria. The immune-enhancing herb echinacea also contains AG, as do leeks, carrots, radishes, pears, wheat, red wine, and tomatoes.

Dosing

Therapeutic Daily Amount: 1000-3000mg per day. A maximum safe level has not been established.

Side Effects/Contraindications: Arabinogalactan may cause bloating. Doses of up to 10 grams per day are seemingly well tolerated. However, very high doses (30 grams or more per day) may cause gastrointestinal side effects. Larch arabinogalactan contains galactose, therefore people with who require a low galactose diet and those with lactose intolerance should avoid taking this supplement. Pregnant women and nursing mothers should avoid larch arabinogalactan supplements.

ASTRAGALUS (ASTRAGALUS MEMBRANACEOUS)

The astragalus or Huang Qi plant hails from China. It has been used in traditional Chinese medicine for more than two thousand years. Astragalus stimulates the adrenal glands, and it is thought that it may help to promote a healthy response to physical and emotional stressors that otherwise could suppress the adrenal glands and lead to sleep difficulties. Astragalus is considered to be a potent immune system booster in Traditional Chinese Medicine. Practitioners report that astragalus reduces the production of T-suppressor cells (cells responsible for terminating the immune response) and increases the activity of T-cells (white blood cells that seek and destroy infectious agents). In turn, astragalus is thought to increase the production of white blood cells in the bone marrow and lymph tissue. Studies performed by the National Cancer Institute and other leading cancer research institutions over have reported that astragalus strengthens the immune system of cancer patients, possibly by increasing the number of white blood cells.

Dosing

Therapeutic Daily Amount: One drop of tincture is taken two to three times per day. The dried root is taken in dosages of 1-4 grams three times per day. Some Chinese Medicine texts recommend taking 9-15 grams of the crude herb per day in decoction form. The most potent astragalus supplements contain a standardized extract of the root, with 0.5% glucosides and 70% polysaccharides. Research suggests that the body can develop a tolerance to immune-stimulating herbs such as astragalus if it is taken for long periods. Therefore some experts recommend alternating astragalus with other immune system-enhancing herbs such as echinacea. A maximum safe level has not been established.

Side Effects/Contraindications: No side effects have been reported. Pregnant women should not take astragalus without consulting their physician first. Astragalus has been found to have a synergistic effect with interferon; therefore those on interferon therapy should discuss whether supplementation with this herb is appropriate. Because some reports have suggested that fresh astragalus contains chemicals known as exudate gums that cause allergic reactions in some people, those with gum allergies should consult a physician before taking this herb.

BLACK CURRANT SEED OIL (RIBES NIGRUM)

In European folk medicine, black currant once had a considerable reputation for controlling diarrhea, promoting urine output (as a diuretic) and reducing arthritic and rheumatic pains. Black currant seed oil is a rich source of gamma-linoleic acid (GLA) and alpha-linoleic acid. Dayong *et al* found that 4.5 g daily of black currant seed oil was able to promote cell-mediated immune function in healthy elderly subjects. The researchers believe that black currant seed oils immune-enhancing effect is attributable to its ability to reduce prostaglandin E (2) (a compound that modifies inflammatory responses) production.

Dosing

Therapeutic Daily Amount: A daily dosage of 600 to 6,000 milligrams is typical. Capsules containing black currant oil are available in 200 to 400 milligram doses – the capsules typically have a fixed oil component, and usually contain 14 to 19% GLA.

Side Effects/Contraindications: No side effects have been reported, however German health authorities warn that people with fluid accumulation, because of heart or kidney problems, should not take the leaf preparations. It should be noted, that no studies appear to have been done to determine the safety of black currant seed extract over the long term, although preliminary findings for other GLA-rich oils suggest that the supplements are relatively safe.

BONESET (EUPATORIUM PERFOLIATUM)

Boneset is indigenous to the Central and Eastern US, and is a popular remedy in Native American Medicine and Traditional Chinese Medicine. Research suggests that boneset has a stimulatory effect upon the immune system. Boneset is especially recommended for the relief of the symptoms that accompany influenza, particularly muscle pain. As well as easing the aches and pains, it can also reduce fever and help to clear mucous from the upper respiratory tract.

Dosing

Therapeutic Daily Amount: Boneset is most commonly found in homeopathic medicines, therefore if you wish to use Boneset it is best to take the advice of a qualified homeopath. However, it is also available, albeit less commonly, in other forms. Recommended doses for the treatment of influenza are: dried herb (1-2g by infusion three times a day); liquid extract (1:1 in 25% alcohol, 1-2 ml three times a day); solid extract (300-500 mg three times a day); tincture (1:5 in 45% alcohol, 1-4 ml three times a day).

Side Effects/Contraindications: Skin contact with the plant itself may cause an allergic reaction. Potential side effects include excessive sweating and diarrhea. High doses may cause vomiting.

CHAMOMILE (MATRICARIA CHAMOMILLA/MATRICARIA RECUTITA)

Chamomile contains active chemical constituents that reduce inflammation, which are responsible for the herb's association as a tea in soothing a sore throat, but also points to its potential usefulness in improving inflammatory conditions such as arthritis and joint problems. Chamomile appears to help stimulate and regulate the immune system. Laskova and Uteshev from Russian State Medical University found that lab animals exposed to heteropolysaccharide (complex carbohydrate molecules) derived from chamomile were more able to resist immune compromise when subjected to physical stress. In follow-up research, Laskova found specifically that the chamomile polysaccharides stimulated key immune cells and increased the sensitivity of immune cells to signals that prompt for their activation.

Dosing

Therapeutic Daily Dose: Chamomile is available as a dried whole herb (to be used as a tea or bath infusion) and in packaged teas, tablets, capsules, concentrated drops, tinctures, and extracts. It is often taken 3-4 times daily between meals as a tea. Standardized extracts containing 1% apigenin and 0.5% volatile oils may also be used. One to two capsules containing 300-400 mg of extract may be taken 3 times daily. Follow dosage directions on labels.

Side Effects/Contraindications: Medicinal chamomile has a low risk of allergic reactions, however Hausen *et al* reported that so-called "chamomile allergy" may actually be the result of the substitution of dog chamomile (which contains the allergenic compound anthecotulide) for the medicinal-grade varieties. Additionally, there is some concern that people who are allergic other plants in the *Asteraceae* family (ragweed, aster and chrysanthemums) may be allergic to chamomile.

CRANBERRY (VACCINIUM MACROCARPON)

Cranberry is a member of the same family as bilberry and is native to North America. Cranberry has long been recommended for people with recurrent urinary tract infections (UTIs).The pro-anthocyanidins present in cranberry prevent E. coli, the most common cause of UTIs and recurrent UTIs, from adhering to the cells lining the wall of the bladder and urinary tract. The berries have also been shown to reduce bacteria levels in the urinary bladder, an action that may help to prevent future infections. Cranberry is recognised as a general immune system-enhancer, due to its high vitamin C content.

Dosing
Therapeutic Daily Amount:
Most tablets and capsules contain dried, unsweetened juice powder or concentrated extract. An average dose is 500 to 1,000mg per day. Unsweetened cranberry juice (available in some health foods stores) is the most potent cranberry drink, but many people find it difficult to get down; sweetened drinks are more palatable. "Cranberry juice drinks" typically contain 10 to 20% juice, whilst "cranberry juice cocktails" typically have 25 to 35% real juice. Some observers have wondered whether these products were too diluted or sugar-laden to have any therapeutic effects but a number of recent studies have found that they can be quite beneficial. For instance, a 1994 study found that 10 ounces per day of commercially available cranberry juice cocktail was almost twice as effective as a placebo in reducing bacteria in urine. When buying the "juice drinks," one will have to drink roughly twice the amount, 20 ounces a day. Results of a study by Stothers revealed that cranberry tablets were twice as cost effective as organic juice for prevention of UTIs.
Side Effects/Contraindications: Ingestion of large amounts (more than 3-4 liters per day) often results in diarrhea and other gastrointestinal symptoms. Therefore, large doses of cranberry should be avoided if one is taking drugs for urinary or kidney problems, or are pregnant or breast-feeding. People taking drugs that affect the kidneys or the urinary tract should consult their doctor before taking supplementary cranberry.

ECHINACEA (ECHINACEA PURPUREA)

An herb native to North America, echinacea is an important component of Native American medicine, traditionally used as both an anti-inflammatory and an antiseptic, especially for skin problems. Echinacea has been shown to boost the immune system, short-circuit colds and flu, fight bacterial and viral infections, lower fever and calm allergic reactions when taken internally. Echinacea increases levels of the antiviral substance interferon. It also increases the production and activity of white blood cells, and helps them move into the circulatory system more quickly. Goel *et al* found that echinacea stimulates alveolar macrophages (a type of white blood cell that protects the body against infection); this finding gives some support for using the herb for the treatment and prevention of upper respiratory tract infections, such as the common cold, which is one of the most popular uses of the herb. Many studies have found that echinacea (when taken at the first sign of a cold for 8 to 10 days) reduces cold symptoms and/or shortens their duration. For example, Lindenmuth *et al* studied 95 people with early symptoms of cold and flu (such as runny nose, scratchy throat, and fever), those who drank 5 to 6 cups of echinacea tea every day for 5 days felt better sooner than those who drank tea without echinacea. Other studies have found that echinacea reduces cold symptoms by roughly 34%. Many people taken echinacea to try prevent a cold or flu by taking the herb throughout cold and flu season or just after exposure to an infection. Despite the popularity of this approach, several studies suggest that it does not work. The consensus seems to be that echinacea may help treat but not prevent the common cold.

Dosing

Therapeutic Daily Dose: Echinacea products vary widely and often include other ingredients such as zinc and goldenseal. There are three different types of Echinacea (*E. purpurea, E. pallida and E. angustifolia*), and various formulations contain different parts of the plant (leaves, flowers, roots). Studies indicate that the best results occur in people who use a liquid or tincture form, rather than a pill or capsule. To treat colds, flu, or upper respiratory tract infections, one of the following should be taken three times a day: 1-2 grams dried root or herb, drunk as tea; 2 to 3 ml of standardized tincture extract; 200 mg of powdered extract containing 4% phenolics; Tincture (1:5): 1-3 ml; Stabilized fresh extract: 0.75 ml.

Side Effects/Contraindications: Echinacea is one of the least toxic herbs around; it is not known to cause any side effects. Allergic reactions are rare, but people who are allergic to any other plants in the compositae family (which includes sunflowers, daisies, and dandelions) should only take a small dose at first. Echinacea should only be taken on an as-needed basis. German health authorities recommend that people should not take echinacea if they have an autoimmune illness, such as lupus (SLE), are HIV-positive, or have progressive systemic diseases, such as tuberculosis and multiple sclerosis. People with liver disease are also advised to avoid Echinacea. It is recommend that no one should take echinacea either internally or externally for more than 8 weeks in a row. If Echinacea is used for an extended period its efficacy may decline and it may actually impair immune function, therefore holidays are recommended. Echinacea may also interfere with immuno-suppressive drugs, and its use is not recommended during pregnancy.

ELDERBERRY (SAMBUCUS NIGRA)

The elderberry has been used for centuries to treat colds and flu. Scientists believe that antioxidant flavonoids found in the elderberry fight viral infection. Elderberry is most commonly used to treat the runny nose and sore throat of the common cold and to help to reduce the fever, muscle pain, and other symptoms of the flu. It is thought that certain compounds in elderberry may help counter the effects of some strains of influenza by binding to the virus and preventing it from attacking cells. An extract from elderberry called Sambucol has proven effective at treating - not preventing - influenza (type A and B). In a study by Zakay-Rones of 60 patients who had been suffering with flu symptoms for 48 hours or less, half the group took 15 ml of Sambucol four times a day for five days, whilst the other half took a placebo. Patients in the Sambucol group had "pronounced improvements" in flu symptoms after just three days, and nearly 90% of patients were completely cured within two to three days. In comparison, the placebo group took at least six days to recover.

Dosing

Therapeutic Daily Amount: Elderberry is available as tinctures, liquid extracts, lozenges, syrups, standardized extract capsules, and throat sprays. Follow dosage directions on labels. For the treatment of flu 15ml of Sambucol four times a day should be taken at the onset of symptoms.

Sid*e Effects/Contraindications:* No adverse reactions to elderberry are known to exist. Raw berries are edible but may cause nausea and vomiting. Herbal products made from the leaves, stems or bark of the elderberry tree should NOT be taken internally as they contain the potentially fatal poison cyanide.

GARLIC (ALLIUM SATIVUM)

Garlic has been renowned for its medicinal properties throughout history. The main active ingredient of garlic is the sulfur compound allicin, produced by crushing or chewing fresh garlic, which in turn produces other sulfur compounds, including ajoene, allyl sulfides, and vinyldithiins. These sulfur compounds, which are found in few other plants, are thought to be responsible for garlic's documented antibacterial (Louis Pasteur confirmed the antibacterial action of the bulb in 1858), antiviral, antifungal, and other healthful properties. Research published in 2001 suggests that allicin, the main active ingredient of garlic, could be useful in the fight against potentially fatal hospital acquired infections. Researchers found that that topical creams containing just 32 parts per million (ppm) of allicin inhibited the growth of 30 different samples of the antibiotic-resistant bacterium methicillin-resistant Staphylococcus aureus (MRSA), and that concentrations of 256 ppm were enough to kill the bacteria. Meanwhile results of a study by Josling revealed that people who took a daily allicin-containing garlic supplement were more than 50% less likely to catch a cold. Furthermore, those taking the supplement that were unlucky enough to catch a cold tended to recover much more quickly and were significantly less likely to become re-infected with the disease.

Dosing

Therapeutic Daily Dose: Garlic is available fresh or juiced, as well as in tablets, capsules, and tinctures. Odor-controlled powders, concentrates, and capsules are popular forms, as are enteric-coated tablets (which have a coating that prevents the destruction of active compounds by stomach acids). Supplement manufacturers are increasingly standardizing their products for desirable garlic compounds (principally one called allicin, but also total sulfur, allin, and S-allyl cysteine), but debate rages on as to which of these compounds are most important and which formulations are most effective. The potency of garlic products may be described in terms of fresh or whole garlic equivalent; an average dose is 1,500 to 1,800mg of fresh garlic equivalent, approximately equal to eating one-half clove of fresh garlic. To fight infection, 3 or 4 chopped, crushed or chewed cloves should be consumed per day or, in supplement form (1.3% allicin), 600–900 mg divided into 2–3 doses/day. Garlic can help to treat colds and flu, however it is best seen as a preventative. The use of garlic against colds and flu seems to be most effective when applied before the infection is caught, or immediately the symptoms begin to show. In Josling's study, which showed that garlic offers protection against the common cold, participants took one capsule of Allimax, an allicin-containing garlic supplement, each day.

Side Effects/Contraindications: Garlic is extremely safe but taking very large daily doses (more than 10g) of some products may cause flatulence, stomach irritation, or indigestion. Because of garlic's anti-clotting properties, persons taking anticoagulant drugs, such as Warfarin and Ticlopidine, should check with their doctor before taking garlic. In addition, people scheduled for surgery should inform their surgeon if they are taking garlic supplements. People taking drugs for the treatment of HIV infection and AIDS should consult their specialist before taking supplementary garlic. Women should avoid taking garlic supplements during pregnancy as laboratory studies suggest that they may cause irregular uterine contractions.

GINSENG – SIBERIAN (ELEUTHEROCOCCUS SENTICOSUS)

Ginseng is available as different species, in different preparations, and different doses. White Ginseng usually refers to untreated ginseng, and is said to be less warm than red Ginseng. Typically red Ginseng is steamed and cured with other herbs giving it a dark red appearance. There are two main kinds of Ginseng, American (Panax quinquefolium) and Asian (Panax Ginseng). American Ginseng has been found of benefit to individuals who are under physical stress (indicating "heat" in Traditional Chinese Medicine [TCM]), such as athletes and people who feel hot and thirsty. Asian Ginseng has been used traditionally to "cold" syndromes (in the TCM system), such as cold limbs, weak pulse, exhaustion, and shortness of breath.

Siberian Ginseng, also known as Eleuthero Ginseng, is really not ginseng at all but is in fact a distant cousin. It belongs in a different botanical species: Eleutherococcus Senticosus. Eleuthero Ginseng grows in northern China, Russia, Korea, and Japan. Although it is used to help the body adapt to stress, it is less specific as a medicinal herb than Asian or American Ginseng. Chemists have isolated more than three-dozen compounds in Siberian ginseng that may affect the mind and body; foremost among these are the eleutherosides, which occur in the plant's roots and, to a lesser degree, in the leaves. Siberian ginseng is known to boost overall immune function and research has shown that compounds found in Siberian ginseng have strong antiviral activity against certain types of viruses, including those that cause the common cold and influenza. Research on mice found that Siberian ginseng enhanced the cellular response of the immune system and boosted antibody production.

Dosing

Therapeutic Daily Dose: Siberian ginseng is sold in capsules, tinctures, and extracts. Standardized Siberian ginseng products often specify the content of one or more of a series of chemicals known as eleutherosides. An average dose is 100-200 mg of an extract standardized for 1% eleutherosides. Siberian ginseng should not be used continuously for more than 6-8 weeks, with a break of 1-2 weeks between use.

Side Effects/Contraindications: Siberian ginseng is considered to be safe for daily consumption even in doses many times larger than average, though some people may experience insomnia and other side effects from taking high amounts. It is recommended that Siberian ginseng should be taken before 3 pm in order to reduce the risk of insomnia. Siberian ginseng should be avoided, or taken with caution, by individuals with uncontrolled high blood pressure and those who are hysteric, manic, or schizophrenic. It should not be taken with stimulants, including coffee, antipsychotic drugs or during treatment with hormones. People taking digoxin should consult their doctor before taking Siberian ginseng.

GOLDENSEAL (HYDRASTIS CANADENSIS)

Goldenseal is native to eastern North America. The dried root and rhizome are used medicinally. With anti-inflammatory and antibiotic properties, the herb goldenseal is effective against bacteria and fungi. The primary active ingredients in goldenseal are the alkaloids hydrastine and berberine, along with smaller amounts of canadine. Berberine, which has been extensively researched, appears to have a wide spectrum of antimicrobial activity against pathogens, including *Chlamydia, E. coli,* and *Salmonella typhi,* as well as viruses and protozoans. Goldenseal is often combined with echinacea in preparations designed to strengthen the immune system. Many herbalists recommend goldenseal in herbal remedies for hay fever, colds, and flu. The herb also appears to stimulate the activity of macrophages (a type of white blood cell that protects the body against infection), the immune cells that attack harmful bacteria, and increase immunoglobulin (proteins used by the immune system to identify and neutralize foreign objects like bacteria and viruses) production.

Dosing
Therapeutic Daily Amount: Standardized extracts supplying 8–12% alkaloids are available; the recommended dose is 30-120 mg three times per day. Goldenseal should not be used continuously for more than 3 weeks, and it recommended that breaks should last at least 2 weeks.
Side Effects/Contraindications: Taken as recommended, goldenseal is generally regarded as safe, however the herb should be avoided during pregnancy and lactation and by those with heart disease, high blood pressure, and diabetes. Some studies have suggested that Goldenseal may reduce the efficacy of doxycycline and tetracycline. Goldenseal may be contraindicated if allergic to ragweed.

GRAPEFRUIT SEED EXTRACT

Grapefruit seed extract (GSE) has a proven track record as a powerful and non-toxic antimicrobial agent with a broad spectrum of activity. GSE can be used in a variety of ways to boost protection against pathogens. Researchers have had positive results using GSE as an antimicrobial agent on food, and as a deep cleanser for skin. Added to toothpaste and mouthwash, GSE may protect against both viral and bacterial infection in the mouth. Some asthmatics have used GSE in nebulizers, reportedly with great success, in order to prevent against lung and bronchial infections.

Dosing

Therapeutic Daily Dose: Refer to dosage information on labels. Be careful not to confuse GSE with "grape seed extract."

Side Effects/Contraindications: Grapefruit seed extract is not associated with any side effects, drug interactions, or contraindications. However, a number of medications should not be taken with grapefruit juice itself. These include certain immunosuppressants, cholesterol-lowering drugs, and antihistamines – if in doubt consult a physician. Furthermore, when taken as recommended it does not destroy the 'healthy' bacteria that reside in the gastro-intestinal tract.

GREEN TEA (CAMELLIA SINENSIS) – A Top Ten Natural Immune Enhancer

Unlike black and oolong tea, green tea is not fermented. This means that the active ingredients remain unaltered in the herb. Green tea contains numerous cancer-fighting polyphenol compounds, including antioxidant flavonoid catechins. The primary catechin in green tea is epigallocatechin gallate (EGCG). Green tea polyphenols are also known to stimulate the production of several immune system cells, and possess antibacterial properties. Drinking green tea may also be a key flu-fighting strategy. Research has shown that drinking green tea stimulates gamma-delta T-cells that boost immunity against viruses. Furthermore, a substance in green tea called L-theanine causes T cells to secrete 10 times their normal output of the virus-fighting interferon. Results of a study by Yamamoto *et al* suggest that EGCG may be a potential immunotherapeutic agent against respiratory infections in immunocompromised patients, such as heavy smokers.

Dosing

Therapeutic Daily Dose: It is possible to buy encapsulated extracts standardized for chemicals called polyphenols. An average dose is 200mg of an extract standardized for 25% polyphenols. An alternative is to buy the dried herb and make tea; which is available in various grades, from twiggy, inexpensive kikich to choice sencha. For maximum benefit, drink up to four or five cups of green tea per day.

Side Effects/Contraindications: The most worrisome chemical in green tea is caffeine, which occurs in small amounts (an average of 20 to 30mg per cup, if brewed for two to three minutes). However, the amount of caffeine in green tea is far lower than that in coffee – an 8-ounce cup of coffee typically contains more than 100mg of caffeine. Unless caffeine has been added, the caffeine content in green tea capsules should be approximately 5 to 15mg. Breastfeeding women are advised to avoid drinking green tea and take supplements instead, as caffeine may have unwanted effects on babies' sleep patterns.

JUJUBE (ZIZYPHYS JUJUBA)

Jujube is a dark red plum-like fruit harvested from trees originally native to northern China. For over 2,000 years, jujube has been a mainstay of Traditional Chinese Medicine. Jujube contains chemical constituents called jujubosides. Matsuda *et al* reported that jujubosides demonstrate potent immune-boosting activity. In China, jujube is used to prevent gastrointestinal and respiratory flu and speed the recovery process.

Dosing

Therapeutic Daily Dose: Take as directed by your practitioner.
Side Effects/Contraindications: Jujube can stimulate the uterus, and therefore pregnant women should not take this supplement.

MUSHROOMS (MAITAKE, SHIITAKE) – A Top Ten Natural Immune Enhancer

Mushrooms are available in a variety of forms, including whole, dried, powdered, tinctures, capsules, tablets, and tea. Known in Japan as the "dancing mushroom," the maitake mushroom is called the "hen of the woods" by American mushroom hunters. An extract from maitake mushrooms called D-fraction is marketed in the US and Japan as a dietary supplement. D-fraction has been shown to stimulate the production of immune cells and increase their effectiveness. Results of a study of D-fraction by Kodama *et al* led the researchers to conclude: "…its administration may enhance host defense against foreign pathogens and protect healthy individuals from infectious diseases." The shiitake (lentinus edodes) mushroom has been revered in Asia for centuries, both as a food and as a medicine. Its most studied active ingredient is the polysaccharide lentinan. Shiitake extract boosts the immune system and combat viruses and bacteria. Shiitake contains vitamins, minerals, amino acids, and a number of polysaccharides, which are linked to countering cancer, primarily by promoting immune function rather than attacking cancer cells directly. Both maitake and shiitake are used traditionally to prevent the common cold and flu.

Dosing

Therapeutic Daily Dose: Maitake: 3-7 grams per day of the supplement is recommended. Maitake mushrooms, fresh or preserved, taste good and can be used in a variety of food preparations. Maitake tea, juice, powder, and granules are available. A liquid extract of maitake D-fraction is available to health professionals. Shiitake: products vary in potency; follow dosage directions on labels.
Side Effects/Contraindications: Maitake: no reported side effects. Shiitake: safe and non-toxic, even in very large doses.

NEEM (AZADIRACHTA INDICA)

More than 140 compounds have been isolated from different parts of the Neem tree. All parts of the tree – leaves, flowers, seeds, fruits, roots and bark have been used medicinally. Neem leaf and its constituents have been demonstrated to exhibit immunomodulatory (capable of modifying or regulating one or more immune functions), anti-inflammatory, antimalarial, antifungal, antiparasitic, antibacterial, antiviral, antioxidant, antimutagenic, and anticarcinogenic properties. In 1855, a researcher reported that Neem leaves were given "with great success" to European soldiers to fight cholera. In 1968, Jain found leaves effective for various skin diseases and boils, and in 1984, Pillai and Santhakumari noted antibacterial action. Recent studies have shown antibiotic efficacy against many bacterial strains, including Staphylococcus and Clostridia. Neem has even successfully healed ulcers associated with bacterial infections.

Neem not only enhances antibody production but also seems to improve the cell-mediated immune response by which white blood cells kill pathogenic organisms. Neem, especially neem bark, is recognized for its immunomodulatory polysaccharide compounds. These compounds appear to increase antibody production. Neem oil acts as a nonspecific immunostimulant that activates the cell mediated immune response. This then creates an enhanced response to any future challenges by disease organisms.

Research by Baral *et al* suggests that Neem leaf preparation (NLP) has immunostimulatory properties. Study results showed that vaccination of mice with both NLP and a melanoma cell surface antigen more efficiently prevented the growth of melanoma tumor than vaccination with the surface antigen or NLP alone. The results led the researchers to conclude: "NLP might be a potential immune adjuvant for inducing active immunity towards tumor antigens."

Dosing
Therapeutic Daily Dose: Refer to packaging.
Side Effects/Contraindications: Numerous studies suggest that leaf and bark are generally regarded as safe, especially when taken orally. Neem oil extracts are considered safe in limited dosage for short periods of time. People who have taken neem oil internally have reported nausea and general discomfort, and excessive consumption of raw neem oil has been implicated in reduced liver functioning. Neem products should not be used by women who are pregnant or breastfeeding.

OLIVE LEAF EXTRACT

A staple of folk medicine for centuries, olive leaves *(Olea europa)* have been used for tea or chopped up as a salad ingredient. Olive Leaf Extract is now recognized for its ability to fight viral and bacterial infections. The plant chemical oleuropein is the source of olive leaf's infection-fighting ability, as it interferes with the production of amino acids that are essential for the survival of bacteria and viruses. Studies have indicated that olive leaf extract can kill the antibiotic-resistant, and potentially fatal, bacteria staphylococcus aureus, and the parainfluenza type 3 virus, which causes a wide range of respiratory illnesses. Due to its anti-vital properties Olive Leaf Extract may also be useful in fighting HIV and AIDS.

Dosing
Therapeutic Daily Dose: Dried leaf extracts containing 6–15% oleuropein are available, however a standard therapeutic amount has not been established.
Side Effects/Contraindications: Olive leaf can irritate the stomach lining; therefore, it should always be taken with meals. Pregnant women should not take olive leaf extract as safety during pregnancy has not yet been established. Olive Leaf Extract may inactivate antibiotics and therefore should not be taken while taking antibiotics.

OPC'S (OLIGOMERIC PROANTHOCYANIDIN COMPLEXES)

Oligomeric proanthrocyanidin complexes, or OPC's, are a specific category of flavonoids. Flavonoids are potent antioxidants that occur naturally in plants and offer them defense against invasions from funguses, toxins, and environmental stress. The richest sources of OPC's are found in red wine extract, grape seed extract, and pine bark extract. The OPC's present in grape seed extract may also help the immune system. Nair *et al* found that grape seed extract promotes the production of interferon (a substance that activates our defenses against viruses) by T-helper 1 cells (a type of white blood cell that helps the body fight off certain infections), thus suggesting that it may help to ward off viral infections. Some of pine barks purported immune boosting and anti-cancer effects may be due to its effect upon macrophages (a type of white blood cell that protects the body against infection). Park *et al* found that found that pine bark extract increases secretion of tumor necrosis factor-alpha (TNF-alpha – a pro-inflammatory chemical messenger that kills tumor cells) by activated macrophages.

Dosing
Therapeutic Daily Dose: The optimal intake of OPC's is yet to be established. Dose will vary depending upon the supplement, thus refer to packaging.
Side Effects/Contraindications: None Known

OREGANO OIL (ORIGANUM VULGARE) – A Top Ten Natural Immune Enhancer

The oil from oregano leaf extract is recommended for the prevention and treatment of a wide range of infectious diseases. Oregano oil is purported to inhibit and/or kill a broad spectrum of pathogenic bacteria, fungi, yeast and protozoal parasites, and some viruses in the gastrointestinal tract. The main active ingredient in oregano oil is carvacrol, however a number of other bioactive monoterpenes, for example thymol, may contribute to its antimicrobial activity. Oregano oil has been scientifically proven to effectively inhibit and/or eliminate a number of pathogens (disease-causing microorganisms), including: *Eschericia coli, Salmonella typhi, Staphylocuccus aureus, Streptococcus pneumoniae, Candida albicans, Cryptococcus neoformans,* and *Giardia lamblia.* It has also been proven that oregano oil is capable of disintegrating the protective membrane of some types of viruses, including Herpes Simplex Virus Type 1, the virus that causes cold sores.

Dosing
Therapeutic Daily Dose: The therapeutic dose of oregano oil ranges between 450 to 1,350 mg per day.
Side Effects/Contraindications: Oregano oil is generally recognized as safe (GRAS). Undiluted oregano oil may cause skin inflammation if applied topically. Oregano oil should not be used by pregnant women.

TEA TREE OIL (MELALEUCA ALTERNIFOLIA)

Tea tree oil is distilled from the leaves of *Melaleuca alternifolia,* a small tree native to Australia. Tea Tree oil is sold as a topical antiseptic and remedy for a whole variety of ailments, including sunburn, sores, cuts, arthritis, bruises, insect bites, warts, acne, fungal infections, mouth ulcers, and dandruff. Tea Tree oil's main infection fighting ingredient is terpinen-4-ol. Terpinen-4-ol weakens bacteria so that the immune system can fight them more effectively, and kills a variety of microbes, including some that conventional antibiotics are ineffective against. *In vitro* (in glass, for example in a test tube) studies have shown that an 0.5% solution of tea tree oil (lower than that found in commercial concentrations) can both inhibit and kill certain antibiotic-resistant bacteria that are common in hospitals, for example the potentially deadly bacteria *Staphylococcus aureus.* Messager *et al* found that a tea tree oil handwash was effective at reducing the activity of *Escherichia coli.* Other studies have shown that the oil is also effective in fighting organisms responsible for vaginal infections, including *Trichomonas vaginalis* and *Candida albicans.*

Dosing
Therapeutic Daily Dose: Tea tree oil is used externally in concentrations of 0.4 to 100%, depending on what part of the body it is applied to and for what purpose. It should not be taken internally.
Side Effects/Contraindications: Tea Tree oil can irritate sensitive skin, however it is generally regarded as safe to use when applied externally. Tea tree oil should never be swallowed as it may cause nerve damage.

FUNCTIONAL/VITAL NUTRACEUTICALS

APPLE CIDER VINEGAR

Apple cider is a natural source of acetic acid. Apple cider vinegar has both antiseptic and antibiotic properties. It is often recommended for relieving the symptoms and congestion of flu, and for treating sore throat, cuts, wounds, digestive problems, and gum infections. There is also some evidence to suggest that Apple Cider vinegar may have the potential to destroy both A and B strains of the human herpes virus-6 (HHV-6).

Dosing
Therapeutic Daily Dose: Refer to packaging. In the event that taking liquid vinegar is cumbersome or inconvenient, vinegar tablets, 500 mg each (equivalent to one tablespoon of liquid vinegar), are available from health food stores. Hill *et al* carried out a study of eight apple cider vinegar tablet products after an adverse event was reported to the authors. The products were tested for pH, component acid content, and microbial growth. Considerable variability was found between the brands in tablet size, pH, component acid content, and label claims. Furthermore, doubt remains as to whether apple cider vinegar was in fact an ingredient in the evaluated products.
Side Effects/Contraindications: None known.

BETA-GLUCAN – 1,3

Beta-glucan is a polysaccharide derived from baker's yeast, young rye plants, and some medicinal mushrooms. Beta-glucan is known to help the immune system fight bacterial, viral, fungal, and parasitic pathogens by activating macrophages (a type of white blood cell that protects the body against infection). Taken before and after surgery, beta-glucan has been shown to help reduce infection. It also appears to enhance the activity of conventional antibiotics.

Dosing

Therapeutic Daily Dose: Most manufacturers recommend doses ranging between 50 and 1,000 mg. However, doses as high as 15,000 mg per day have been used to lower cholesterol in clinical trials. A maximum safe level has not been established.
Side Effects/Contraindications: None known.

BEE PRODUCTS

Bees produce several substances that are useful to humans, these are: honey, propolis, pollen, and royal jelly. Research shows that honey can stimulate the immune system and help the body to deal with infections by activating immune cells. Used as a skin treatment, honey prevents infection and speeds healing by starving existing bacteria and protecting the skin from infection by new bacteria. Research by Natarajan *et al* suggests that honey could prove useful in the fight against antibiotic-resistant "superbugs" such as MRSA. Propolis is rich in anti-inflammatory and antioxidant flavonoids. It also contains terpenoids, which have antibacterial, antiviral, antiprotozoan, and antifungal effects. Research by Takagi et al showed that propolis stimulates the immune system in a number of ways, including activating macrophages (a type of white blood cell that protects the body against infection) and increasing the proliferation of T-cells (white blood cells that are crucial to the immune system) white blood cell crucial to the immune system). For acute internal infections, propolis can be taken along with regularly prescribed medications. Bee pollen contains a wealth of nutrients utilized by the human body, including vitamins, minerals, enzymes, and amino acids. Royal jelly contains several vitamins and is thought to have anti-inflammatory properties. Studies suggest that royal jelly may also have potent immunomodulatory (capable of modifying or regulating one or more immune functions) properties both in vitro (in glass, for example in a test tube) and in vivo (in the body).

Dosing

Therapeutic Daily Dose: Refer to packaging.
Side Effects/Contraindications: Pollen: Bee pollen should not be taken during pregnancy. Propolis: Allergic reactions to topically applied propolis are quite common, typically they involve pain, redness, swelling, and sores. Use should be discontinued straight away. Propolis is also a known "sensitizing agent," therefore regular use can cause people to develop allergies to the product. Royal Jelly: Contraindicated during pregnancy.

BROMELAIN (PINEAPPLE ENZYME)

Bromelain is a proteolytic enzyme (an enzyme that digests proteins) found in fresh pineapple. It is often used to treat muscle injuries and as a digestive aid. There is evidence to suggest that bromelain may enhance immune function. Barth *et al* found that bromelain activates macrophages (a type of white blood cell that protects the body against infection) and has positive effects on other factors. The results of the study led the authors to conclude: "…[bromelain] may stimulate, therefore, the innate as well as the adaptive immune system." Other research has shown that bromelain also activates natural killer cells (a type of white blood cell that destroys tumor cells and cells infected with certain organisms). When applied topically it may help to speed wound healing. Bromelain may also enhance the effect of the antibiotics amoxicillin, erythromycin, penicillamine, and penicillin. In a study of people with urinary tract infections, 100% of participants given antibiotics in combination with bromelain and another enzyme called trypsin were cured of their infection, compared with just 46% who received antibiotics alone.

Dosing
Therapeutic Daily Amount: Bromelain is measured in MCUs (milk clotting units) or GDUs (gelatin dissolving units), where one GDU equals roughly 1.5 MCU. Potent bromelain products contain approximately 2,000 MCU per gram. Some doctors recommend taking up to 3,000 MCU thrice daily for several days, and then decreasing the dosage to three daily 2,000 MCU doses.

Side Effects/Contraindications: Bromelain is generally regarded as being safe and side effect-free when taken as directed. However, some people may be allergic to bromelain as it is derived from pineapple. Bromelain is not recommended for people with active gastric or duodenal ulcers. People taking anticoagulant drugs such as warfarin should not take supplementary bromelain without consulting their physician.

COD LIVER OIL (FISH OIL)

As its name suggests, cod liver oil is oil extracted from cod livers. Cod liver oil is one of the best sources of the essential omega-3 fatty acids DHA (docosahexaenoic acid) and EPA (eicosapentaenoic acid), and is a rich source of vitamins A and D. Cod liver oil and fish oil are similar but have a somewhat different composition: fish oil has a much lower content of vitamins A and D compared to liver oils. Omega-3 fatty acids have profound anti-inflammatory effects when taken at a therapeutic dosage. Omega-3's help curb an overactive immune system and thus are helpful in the treatment of autoimmune diseases such as rheumatoid arthritis, chronic inflammatory bowel disease, Crohn's disease, and psoriasis. Omega-3's are also effective in curbing the inflammatory response to severe burns, sepsis, systemic inflammatory response syndrome (SIRS) and asthma. Nordvik *et al* found that omega-3's can improve the clinical outcome for newly diagnosed multiple sclerosis patients. Omega-3's may confer greater resistance to common illnesses such as influenza and the common cold.

Dosing

Therapeutic Daily Dose: The majority of research into the effects of DHA and EPA in humans have used doses of at least 3g of DHA plus EPA supplements. To obtain a similar amount of DHA and EPA from fish oil it may be necessary to consume as much as 10g, as most fish oils contain only 18% EPA and 12% DHA. It is important to buy a good quality, mercury-free, cod liver oil/fish oil supplement. A maximum safe dose has not established. Burns *et al* found that the maximum amount of fish oil tolerated by people being treated for cancer-related weight loss was roughly 21g per day. However, the maximum tolerated amount in people without cancer may well be different. High doses of fish oil (3 g and above) should only be taken if directed to do so by an expert.

Side Effects/Contraindications: Cod liver oil should be used cautiously by people who have a bleeding disorder, or take blood-thinning medications as excessive amounts of omega-3 fatty acids may lead to bleeding. People who consume more than three grams of omega-3 fatty acids per day (equivalent to 3 servings of fish per day) may be at an increased risk for hemorrhagic stroke.

COLLOIDAL SILVER

Often called the "penicillin of alternative medicine," colloidal silver (CS) is said to disable the enzymes that bacteria, parasites, viruses, and fungi rely on to use oxygen, therefore killing the pathogens. However, there is little scientific evidence to support these claims. Among the conditions CS has reportedly controlled are severe burns, acne, boils, candida and yeast infections, chronic fatigue syndrome, digestive problems and colitis, ear and sinus infections, herpes, shingles, lupus, malaria, viral and fungal infections, blood parasites, rheumatoid arthritis, and ringworm. CS also has been reported to be effective in treating cancer and AIDS, however these uses of CS are not clinically proven.

Dosing

Therapeutic Daily Dose: The recommended dosage of CS depends upon the concentration of the product. Concentration of CS is expressed as "ppm" or "parts per million." Concentrations range from 5ppm to 500ppm. In general, the greater the ppm the larger the CS particle size. This variable is important because it takes a smaller particle size to kill a virus than it does to kill bacteria. Some companies have developed technology that allows increased ppm while preserving a smaller particle size. CS can be taken internally in a small amount of distilled drinking water. It also can be applied topically to cuts and open sores. Nebulization of CS, which delivers colloidal silver directly into the lung tissues and bloodstream, is a highly effective way to use colloidal silver; by bypassing the digestive system, some believe that a greater amount of colloidal silver can be delivered into the body. However, this should only be done under the direct supervision of a medical professional, as when colloidal silver carrying mist reaches infected lung tissues, it can cause pain and difficulty breathing.

Side Effects/Contraindications: Clinical research has uncovered no adverse effects from properly prepared colloidal silver, nor have there been any reported cases of CS-drug interaction. CS should not be used for prolonged periods of time (more than seven consecutive days). Note: In February 1997, the US Food and Drug Administration (FDA) issued the following statement: "The use of colloidal silver-containing products constitutes a potentially serious public health concern … the consumption of silver by humans may result in argyria – a permanent ashen-gray or blue discoloration of the skin, conjunctiva (white of the eye), and internal organs." Argyria is not treatable or reversible, and is thought to result from products containing high concentrations of silver compounded with stabilizers such as silver nitrate or silver acetate. Argyria has never been reported from pure electro-colloidal silver free of protein or other stabilizers. Over-the-counter colloidal silver products are not considered by the US FDA to be generally recognized as safe (GRAS) and effective for diseases and conditions. Colloidal silver-containing products have never been approved by the FDA for treatment of any disease in any animal species.

COLOSTRUM (BOVINE)

Within hours of giving birth, human and animal mothers secrete colostrum as a prelude to breast milk. Colostrum gives newborns a "vaccination" of antibodies, immune system protection, and growth factors. Whole colostrum is preferred over defatted colostrum because fat is necessary to assist in transporting colostrum protein into the bloodstream. Colostrum is primarily taken for its immune system enhancing benefits. Crooks *et al* studied the effects of bovine (cow) colostrum on athletes. Results showed that supplementation with bovine colostrum for twelve weeks led to a 79% increase in levels of secretory IgA (an immunoglobulin (a protein that acts as an antibody) found in body fluids such as tears and saliva that protects the body's mucosal surfaces from infection) in saliva. Secretory IgA offers protection against upper respiratory tract infection (URTI). Thus, suggesting that bovine colostrum may be of benefit to people at risk of URTIs, such as influenza, and the common cold.

Dosing

Therapeutic Daily Dose: manufacturers often recommend 1,000 to 4,000 mg per day of freeze-dried colostrum. Colostrum is now available in capsules that contain its immune proteins in dry form.

Side Effects/Contraindications: No significant side effects of colostrums have been reported.

INOSITOL HEXAPHOSPHATE (IP6) – A Top Ten Natural Immune Enhancer

Inositol hexaphosphate is a naturally occurring component of plant fiber that is thought to possess antioxidant, anticancer, and other beneficial properties. IP6 is found in the germ of bran portion of whole grains (especially whole kernel corn) and legumes. IP6 enhances the immune system by boosting the activity of natural killer cells (a type of white blood cell that destroys tumor cells and cells infected with certain organisms). IP6 is also thought to prevent tumor development by controlling cell development, and may assist in the treatment of existing cancer by helping natural killer cells to enter cancer cells and by triggering cancer cells to undergo apoptosis (cellular suicide).

Dosing
Therapeutic Daily Amount: A typical dose of IP6 as a preventive supplement is 1-2 g/day. Higher doses are used for the treatment of cancer, however if used for this reason, IP6 should only be taken under the direction of a qualified health professional.
Side Effects/Contraindications: IP6 can interfere with iron absorption, thus it should only be taken under medical supervision. People with cancer or immune-related illnesses should talk to their specialist before taking IP6.

ISOFLAVONES

Soy-based foods such as soymilk, tempeh, and tofu, contain potent compounds called isoflavones that are chemically similar to the female hormone estrogen. Many scientists believe that the widespread use of soy in Eastern diets may help to explain why the incidence of hormone-related cancers is much lower among Asian women. Numerous studies suggest that the soy isoflavone genistein may actually suppress the immune system. Results of a study in mice by Yellayi *et al* showed that when mice were injected with genistein levels of several immune system cells dropped, and the thymus, a gland where T-cells mature (white blood cells that are crucial to the immune system), shrank. However, more alarmingly, the thymus also shrank when mice were fed genistein in their diet. The authors of this study recommend that soy intake should be limited to no more than roughly

100mg a day. Studies have also found evidence to suggest that feeding babies soy-based infant formulas increases their risk of autoimmune disease later in life. However, there is also animal research to suggest that genistein stimulates various aspects of immune function. In conclusion, more work is needed to definitively establish the effects that genistein has on the immune system.

Dosing

Therapeutic Daily Dose: No maximum safe level of soy isoflavones has been established, however some experts recommend that soy intake should be limited to no more than 100mg a day.

Side Effects/Contraindications: In laboratory studies, soy has been shown to stimulate the growth of breast cells, whether or not this increases the risk of breast cancer remains unclear, and research is ongoing. However, women with a medical history or family history of breast cancer are advised to consult their doctor before taking soy isoflavone supplements. Several groups of people should avoid taking soy isoflavone supplements, these include: pregnant women, nursing women, women trying to conceive, and people taking estrogens, ipratropium bromide, thyroid hormones, or warfarin.

LACTOBACILLUS ACIDOPHILUS

Lactobacillus acidophilus is a "friendly" strain of bacteria, which colonises the intestines where it helps prevent intestinal infections. Lactobacillus also flourishes in the vagina, where it protects women against yeast infections. Along with other "friendly" microbes, Lactobacillus is known as a "probiotic". There is evidence that *Lactobacillus acidophilus* may help to strengthen the immune system. Results of a study by Sheih *et al* led the authors to conclude:"[*Lactobacillus acidophilus*] appears to enhance systemic cellular immune responses and may be useful as a dietary supplement to boost natural immunity." The primary dietary sources of Lactobacillus acidophilus include: milk enriched with acidophilus, yogurt containing live Lactobacillus acidophilus cultures, miso, and tempeh.

Dosing

Therapeutic Daily Dose: A typical daily dose of *Lactobacillus* should supply about 3-5 billion live organisms.

Side Effects/Contraindications: Immunocompromised people should consult their doctor before taking probiotics.

The World Health Network
www.worldhealth.net
The Official Website of the American Academy of
   Anti-Aging Medicine (A4M)
The Internet's Leading Anti-Aging Portal

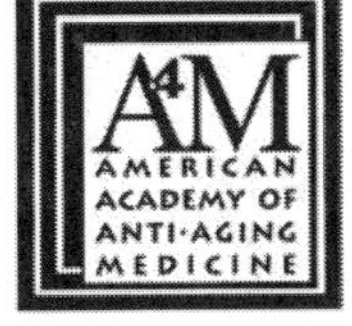

LACTOFERRIN – A Top Ten Natural Immune Enhancer

Lactoferrin is a protein found in breast milk, which helps the infant to combat infection whilst the immune system is not yet fully functional. Lactoferrin is most abundant in colostrum. Lactoferrin regulates iron in the digestive tract, thus helping to maintain the balance of helpful bacteria and harmful bacteria that need iron to grow. Lactoferrin is thought to boost the immune system. Research has shown that lactoferrin modulates the migration, maturation, and function of immune cells. Artym *et al* found that lactoferrin helped to accelerate the restoration of immune responsiveness in bone marrow transplant recipients whose immune systems' had been impaired by chemotherapy. Lactoferrin has both antibacterial and antiviral properties. Research has shown that it may be useful for the treatment of HIV when taken in combination with standard antiretrovital therapy.

Dosing
Therapeutic Daily Dose: Refer to packaging.

PLANT STEROLS (SAPONINS)

Saponins are a group of plant chemicals found in found in soybeans, chickpeas, asparagus, tomatoes, potatoes, and oats. In nature, saponins appear to act as antibiotics that protect plants from microbes. In humans, saponins might fight cancer and infection. Research supports the use of saponins as adjuvants (an additional treatment used to increase the effectiveness of the primary therapy) to enhance the immune response to vaccines. Several *in vitro* (in glass, for example in a test tube) and *in vivo* (in the body) studies have found evidence to support the belief that saponins have potent anticarcinogenic properties. It is thought that saponins protect against cancers via a range of different mechanisms, including an overall antioxidant effect, direct and select cytotoxicity of cancer cells, immune-modulation, and regulation of cell proliferation.

Dosing
Therapeutic Daily Dose: Depends upon preparation – refer to packaging. It is extremely important not to exceed the recommended dosage, as saponins are highly toxic.
Side Effects/Contraindications: The majority of saponins cause some degree of bloating. They can also cause nausea and diaarhea. Pregnant women and people who are anemic or who have other blood disorders should not take saponins without consulting their doctor.

TRANSFER FACTORS

HS Lawrence discovered transfer factors in 1949, when he found that the immune fraction of an individual's white blood cells was able to transfer immunity to a non-sensitized person. As small messenger molecules, transfer factors conduct immune recognition signals between immune cells. In doing so, they help "educate" young immune cells about present or potential danger. The most abundant source of transfer factors is colostrum, the "first milk" of humans and other animals such as cows. Transfer factors have been used to treat bacterial and viral infections, parasites, and fungal disease. Research has shown that transfer factors are effective in treating chronic sinusitis, viral hepatitis, chronic candidiasis, chronic infection, otitis media, AIDS, other viral infections. There is also evidence to suggest that transfer factors may be useful in the treatment of certain types of cancer. A deficiency of transfer factors may leave a person vulnerable to infection.

Dosing

Therapeutic Daily Dose: Standard transfer factors, use for preventive purposes, are balanced preparations with no one factor predominating. Refer to dosage instruction on packaging or use as directed by a physician.
Side Effects/Contraindications: Transfer factors may cause flu-like symptoms in some individuals.

WHEY PROTEIN

As a derivative of milk production, the amino acids in whey proteins are closely related to the amino acids required by the human body. Whey is thought to help boost the immune system, fight infection, and help the body recover from stress. Whey protein contains approximately 2.5% cysteine, which is known to increase the cellular level of the potent antioxidant glutathione. Glutathione plays an important role in the regulation of immune cells and may possess antiviral properties. Whey also contains the protein lactoferrin, which is known to boost the immune system and modulate the migration, maturation, and function of immune cells. Van Dissel *et al* treated 16 patients with a history of relapsing *Clostridium difficile* diarrhoea. Results showed that just two weeks of treatment with whey proteins removed all traces of the bacteria from the faeces of all but one participant. When participants were followed-up one year later, none had suffered another bout of *Clostridium difficile* – associated diarrhoea.

Dosing

Therapeutic Daily Dose: Most people should not need to take supplementary whey protein, as they should obtain enough protein from their diet. However, people who have undergone recent trauma, surgery, and those who participate in strenuous exercise may benefit from taking up to 25g of whey protein per day. Of the various forms available (concentrate, peptides, hydrolysate, etcetera) whey protein isolate is considered superior by many because of its purity, high glutathione content and increased bioavailability.

Side Effects/Contraindications: Whey may be contraindicated in people with milk allergies. Long-term, excessive intake of whey protein, as with other proteins, is not recommended, as it may be associated with deteriorating kidney function and possibly osteoporosis.

OTHER NUTRIENTS

EPICOR™ – A Top Ten Natural Immune Enhancer

EpiCor™ is a new dietary supplement with remarkable potential for health protection and maintenance of the immune system. Not an herb or an isolated nutrient, EpiCor is the product of a sophisticated fermentation process that creates a whole food concentrate with high levels of nutritional metabolites and exceptionally powerful antioxidant and immune modulating activity.

Scientifically documented research demonstrates that EpiCor™ acts multi-modally to confer the following properties:

- Antimicrobial activity: EpiCor™ significantly inhibits the growth of *E. coli* and *Candida tropicalis*, even at concentrations as low as 1 part per trillion. Not only does EpiCor™ inhibit the growth of undesirable, pathogenic bacteria & fungus, but given the proper growth environment (such as in the human body), this could encourage the growth of favorable bacterial organisms in the gut whose secondary metabolites contribute to human health.

- Improves CD4/CD8 T-cell ratio: CD4 (helper) cells facilitate and coordinate immune response, while CD8 (suppressor) cells, in part, down-regulate this response. So a higher ratio of CD4 to CD8 cells is desirable for mounting an effective immune response. EpiCor™ produces a significant reduction in the levels of CD8 cells and produces a more favorable CD4/CD8 ratio. This results in increased antibody production and pathogen-killing activity *in vitro*. As it turns out, blood samples taken from persons ingesting EpiCor™ daily found they had significantly better helper to suppressor (CD4:CD8) cell ratios than their age- and gender- matched counterparts.

- Activates natural killer (NK) cells: EpiCor™ increases NK cell activity by fourfold *in vitro*. NK cells are the most aggressive of your body's immune cells and are among the most important in controlling viral proliferation. NK cells' sole mission is to destroy abnormal cells and those infected with viruses such as SARS, West Nile and Avian Flu. One reason that NK cells are so crucial to viral protection is that, when they identify an infected cell, they destroy it by inducing apoptosis (cell death) rather that by merely dismantling the cell membrane. This is a crucial distinction because apoptosis also destroys the viral particles inside the infected cell, whereas lysing the cell membrane would only release parasitic viral fragments to spread further. Blood samples taken from persons ingesting EpiCor™ daily found they had significantly more efficient NK cells than their age- and gender- matched counterparts.

- <u>Increases levels of salivary Secretory IgA (sIgA):</u> Immnoglobulins (Ig) are a family of antibodies found throughout the body. Secretory IgA (sIgA) is found on the mucosal surfaces of the body like the gastrointestinal tract, nasal passages, and eyes, where it forms the first line of defense against bacteria, viruses and other pathogens. Since deactivation at the point of entry is an exceptionally efficient anti-viral and anti-bacterial strategy, keeping sIgA levels at optimal levels is a good idea. Supplementation with EpiCor™ produced very high sIgA levels (over 300 mg per ml) in persons consuming EpiCor™. This is the equivalent of an immunological "envelope" protecting those membranes in the body where pathogenic organisms might enter into the system.
- <u>Reduces interferon-gamma levels:</u> Interferon-gamma is a marker of inflammation, which plays an adverse contributory role to the severity of respiratory diseases including influenza A and bird flu.

The EpiCor™ Story

EpiCor™ was first discovered over sixty years ago. In the plant in which it is manufactured, production workers appeared to gain immunity by merely inhaling small amounts of EpiCor™ each day, part of which was ingested and digested in the gut. An initial oxygen radical absorbance capacity (ORAC) assay (a measure of antioxidant activity) revealed that EpiCor™ possessed the second highest peroxyl radical scavenging activity (610 μmoleTE/g) of any food ever tested. Additional antioxidant assays discovered that EpiCor™ had even broader free radical scavenging activity *in vitro* against not only the peroxyl radical but also for both the hydroxyl and peroxynitrite radicals, which is unusual for an antioxidant found in the diet.

In addition, the workers at the plant who were "exposed" to EpiCor™ daily were able to fight off infectious agents circulating at their place of employment or in the community at large. So even when a flu epidemic occurred in the community, their immune system responded so effectively, that it kept them out of bed, and thereby avoiding the need to call in sick.

Dosing

Therapeutic Daily Dose: One 500 mg capsule daily or as directed by your health care practitioner. The immunomodulatory effects become clinically evident after 2 1/2 weeks of daily consumption.

Side Effects/Contraindications: The results of all the studies completed to date indicate that EpiCor is safe, non-toxic, non-mutagenic, non-mitogenic, non-cytotoxic, pesticide free and regarded as Generally Recognized as Safe (GRAS) by the FDA.

EpiCor™ is available from a company called Vitamin Research Products (www.vrp.com).

IMMUNOMAX — A Top Ten Natural Immune Enhancer

ImmunoMax is a safe and effective botanical formulation composed of the medicinal herbs:

- Astragalus membranaceus, root, as an extract containing seventy percent (70%) polysaccharides;
- Andrographis paniculata, providing ten percent (10%) andrographolidess and neoandrographolide;
- and the two varieties of Purple Coneflower - Echinacea angustifolia, contributing four percent (4%) echinacosides, plus Echinacea purpura, containing eight percent (8%) total polyphenols.

This synergistic product provides immune support, and has been designed to ameliorate the duration and severity of upper respiratory infections (U.R.I.).

ImmunoMax works to:

- Support and enhance the effectiveness of both systemic and local immune defenses
- Reduce the duration and severity of a wide spectrum infections caused by viruses, bacteria and fungi
- Provide support to the 'Antioxidant Defense System'
- Protect the liver and re-establish homeostatic immunomodulatory benefits
- Enhance the effectiveness of antiviral compounds
- Minimize the cytotoxic side effects of drugs

Dosing

Recommended Amount: One capsule three times daily or as recommended by your health care professional.

Side Effects/Contraindications: Because ImmunoMax enhances immune function, it should not be taken by transplant recipients or individuals who have autoimmune conditions. It is not recommended for pregnant or nursing women.

According to Varro Tyler's Herbs of Choice, Echinacea should not be used by those suffering from severe, chronic systemic illnesses. Germany's Commission E, a government-established committee to determine safety and efficacy of herbal remedies, recommends that use of Echinacea should not exceed a period of eight successive weeks.

ImmunoMax is produced by a company called Vitamin Research Products (www.vrp.com).

ALKALINE WATER

Alkaline water is water with a pH balance of more than 7.4. Alkaline water is also said to balance the body's pH, which is often acidic, especially in people who are ill. The Western lifestyle and diet is said to leave a lot of acidic waste in the body, which can build up over time and create an ideal environment for diseases and cancer cells to thrive. Drinking alkaline water is said to help the body to maintain an environment that is not conducive to disease. Some say it can also destroy pathogens, such as bacteria and viruses, and support the immune system. The Japanese have been drinking alkaline water since the early 1950s, and in January 1966 alkaline-water making devices were approved as medical devices by the Health and Rehabilitation Department of the Japanese Government. Solutions and water ionizers are available to make water alkaline.

Dosing

Therapeutic Daily Dose: Drinking several glasses of alkaline water a day allegedly helps to remove acidic waste products from the body and restore the pH balance of the body to a more alkaline state.
Side Effects/Contraindications: None known.

OZONATED WATER

Ozone (O_3) consists of three atoms of oxygen bound together, instead of the normal two in oxygen (O_2). Ozone is created artificially as the result of ultraviolet light acting on oxygen to break up and recombine as threesomes. Ozone destroys algae, viruses, bacteria, and fungi on contact. Ozone has potent disinfectant properties, and ozonated water is reportedly very good at killing viruses, such as those that cause flu, if taken within 15 to 30 minutes of adding the ozone to water. A machine is needed to make ozonated water. Smaller, less expensive machines use ultraviolet radiation and air, and such units will take 10-15 minutes to produce one glass of water. More expensive machines use bottled oxygen and a high voltage corona arc to produce ozone, and will produce a glass of ozonated water in 2-3 minutes.

Dosing

Therapeutic Daily Dose: For the treatment of infection, such as influenza, drink one glass of ozonated water every 2-4 hours (for best results drink on an empty stomach) throughout the day until the infection has passed.
Side Effects/Contraindications: Ozonated water can cause nausea.

PROCEDURES

ALKALINIZATION

The Western lifestyle and diet is said to leave a lot of acidic waste in the body, which can build up over time and create an ideal environment for diseases and cancer cells to thrive. The ph of the blood at birth is 7.44, which is alkaline. As we get older acidic waste accumulates and the pH of the blood drops to 7.35 or below, and this can cause a number of problems. A healthy urine is 6.4 to 6.8 on a first-morning void. Healthy pH for saliva should range from 6.4-6.8.

The goal of alkalinization is to restore the body's pH to the alkaline range. Alkalinization is said to help the body to maintain an environment that is not conducive to disease. Some say alkalinization can also destroy pathogens, such as bacteria and viruses, and support the immune system.

Treatment Protocol

The first step in alkalinization is to determine the body's pH by testing the urine with ph paper. Various steps can be taken to restore the body's pH to the alkaline range, these include: drinking alkaline water, eating plenty of vegetables, legumes, and grains, drinking water with a squeeze of fresh lemon juice, taking calcium and magnesium supplements. Fruits are generally sweet, and therefore acidic, thus when following an alkaline diet it is necessary to eat low-sugar (low-glycemic index) fruits, such as tomatoes, avocados, lemons, and limes.

Side Effects/Contraindications

None known.

ESSENTIAL OILS

When administered properly, in many cases essential oils can be an effective alternative to antibiotic drugs. Essential oils are some of the most powerful antibacterial agents known. Certain oils, for example bay laurel and ginger, are thought to have immune system boosting properties. Essential oil therapy has been part of the mainstream European healthcare system for 120 years. Medicinally applied pure essential oils are extremely beneficial in every area of health and complement all healthcare treatments. It is important to use pure, unadulterated essential oils that have not been stored in clear glass, or near light or heat. Essential oil therapy has some contraindications and must be administered responsibly, but essential oils have no toxic side effects and are generally broad-spectrum, that is, they benefit multiple areas of the body at once. Essential oils attack the whole pathogen, not just a specific aspect of the organism. This is commonly thought to be the reason why pathogens do not become resistant to the effects of essential oils.

Treatment Protocol

Medicinal essential oils are delivered by a trained and licensed expert. He or she will instruct you on proper application via inhalation, skin application, and baths.

Side Effects/Contraindications

Certain oils can cause irritation to body tissues and organs. Certain oils are contraindicated in specific diseases and in pregnancy. Consult a knowledgeable Aroma/Essential Oil Therapist prior to using essential oils as a therapeutic intervention.

Expert Insight: "Back to Basics" with Essential Oils

Ms. Anne Vermilye, MSAT, CCHT, CMT has a complementary medical private practice in Mill Valley and Sonoma, California and has been using essential oils along with hypnotherapy and various types of body work for the past 15+ years. She is president and CEO of Bio Excel, LLC, essential oil importers and product formulators. She shares some of her knowledge of this subject with our readers in this interview.

Dr. Ronald Klatz: What is an essential oil, what makes essential plant oils effective, how do they work?

Ms. Anne Vermilye: Essential oils are derived from all parts of the plant-roots, stems, leaves, flowers, seeds and bark. Essential oils are extracted and collected through different processes of distillation. They are effective therapeutically for three reasons, namely: 1) Small molecules allowing them to enter the body's tissues, organs and fluids, even crossing the blood/brain barrier easily; 2) Essential oils are simply and naturally the original pharmacy with the biochemical structures left whole, like they are intended to be used, they are at full strength. Using the oils therapeutically is just getting "back to the basics"; and 3) Essential oils have hundreds of different types of molecules, having effects in multiple areas of the body at the same time. Each essential oil often gives numerous benefits.

RK: The majority of our readers associate aromatherapy with the relaxation response, yet you have scientific evidence as to the potent infection-fighting potential of essential oils. Please tell us about some research study findings.

AV: Infectious diseases are on the rise in every part of the world and many strains are rapidly, even hourly, becoming resistant to standard antibiotics and first line drug treatments. So far, when certain essential oils have been laboratory and clinically tested on some of the antibiotic strains of infections they seem to be very effective against them. In a

(continued)

Expert Insight with Ms. Anne Vermilye *(continued)*

study performed by University of California (Irvine, California USA) researchers, and published in the Summer 2003 issue of the *Journal of the American Nutriceutical Association*, the report titled "Antimicrobial Effects of Plant-Derived Essential Oil Formulations on Pathogenic Bacteria" explains how two plant-derived proprietary essential oil blends were tested for their antibacterial activity against five common strains of pathogenic bacteria. An essential oil formulation intended for topical use inhibited the growth of *Escherichia coli, Klebsiella pneumoniae,* and *Staphylococcus aureus;* a second formulation, for inhalation use, inhibited the growth of all five test bacteria strains, with its inhibition activity demonstrated to be significantly greater than that reported for standard antibiotics.

In a National Institutes of Health Research Report on "Essential Plant Oil Blends versus SARS," published in February 2004, researchers deemed that administration for 48 weeks of a formulation composed of essential oils of cinnamon, tea tree, lavender, rosemary, eucalyptus r., thyme and peppermint, used internally (under the guidance of a trained Aroma/Essential Oil Therapist), as a safe and well tolerated choice for infection (as compared to treatment with interferon).

RK: What are the common ways to use essential oils?
AV: Inhalation, dermal application, baths, oral care, ingestion, rectal and vaginal suppositories are efficient ways to use essential oils. Some methods are better than others depending on what effect is desired and where in the body you want to reach. Essential oils are composed of very small molecules that, when applied to the skin, are readily absorbed. Inhalation introduces essential oils into the body via breathing the vapors as they evaporate and are released into the air. The internal use of essential oils should only be explored after consulting with a knowledgeable Aroma/Essential Oil Therapist, as some oils can irritate sensitive tissue and organs.

RK: What are some do's and don'ts about using essential oils?
AV: First, take care if you have allergies, especially to needle trees, and secondly, do not put irritating oils undilluted on the skin or into bath water. In addition, more does not mean better; a little goes a long way. Women who are pregnant should be careful in using essential oils: there are some super oils to use during pregnancy and the birthing process, but some oils are toxic to fetuses (for example the high ketone content oils sage and juniper).

RK: What about using essentials oils in a healthcare setting?
AV: Healthcare practitioners who use essential oils are positively effected on many levels and feel they are more protected from the germs that are usually brought into the office. For patient care, essential oils have been used successfully to treat antibiotic resistant infections, wounds, ulcers, respiratory and digestion issues, pain management, chronic internal bleeding, edema and depression.

FEVER (HYPERTHERMIA, PYREXIA)

Some medical experts believe that body's fever mechanism has evolved over millions of years as an adaptive response to infection and as such is one of the body's most powerful defenses against disease. In fact, the use of heat for healing – where a body temperature above 98.6°F (37°C) is deliberately induced, a process knows as hyperthermia – is clearly documented in human history. Over 5000 years ago, Egyptians immersed people in hot oil, and the use of hot springs was first documented in the Book of Genesis in the Bible. Hyperthermia has been shown to lower disease and death rates in animals with bacterial and viral infections. Consequently, researchers are taking a close look at hyperthermia as a treatment for HIV/AIDS. The therapy is not without controversy. Some researchers have successfully treated infection by raising the body temperature of patients as high as 106°F (41.1° C) (with 100% humidity) for 10 hours; in other studies, however, some patients have experienced severe side effects and even death. Current proponents of hyperthermia suggest that the maximum safe level of fever not requiring treatment is 103°F (39.4°C); viral replication is inhibited at temperatures at or above 101°F (38.3°C).

Expert Insight: The Public's "Oversensitivity to Fever"

Mr. Fintan Dunne is a technical and medical journalist and editor of MyLongLife.com (www.mylonglife.com). He has written on medical issues as diverse as HIV/AIDS, SARS, and the social psychology of medicine. The following is an excerpt from an interview conducted by Dr. Ronald Klatz with Mr. Dunne; you are invited to visit www.worldhealth.net/pandemic to listen to the entire interview.

Dr. Ronald Klatz: I read on your web site about the folly in trying to defeat a fever when in fact it is the first line of the defense, one of the very early lines of defense of the body against viral infection.

Mr. Fintan Dunne: Let's take you back to the so called big one back in 1918 the Spanish flu, which came around the same time as aspirin became popular. Aspirin, it uncouples oxygen phosphorylization, inhibits lymphocyte transformation, and inhibits interferon production; we now know these are all vital elements of the antiviral response of the body. It's not the only one — other similar products, like the modern analgesics ibuprofen and acetaminophen, they also suppress the production of antibodies and they prolong symptoms. Research shows that if you've got something that lasts 9 days, take these kinds of things; if you've got something that lasts 5 days you don't. It's crazy that we take these things trying to alleviate the short-term symptoms when it's in our best long-term interests to suffer. Some would say "suffer quickly, you'll get rid of it even faster." There is evidence that sweat lodges found in Norwegian and American Indian culture helped to raise the temperature. If you raise the temperature, you boost — your body's immune system works better, so that's a good start. So the body also cuts back on sugar production, so don't interfere with that — it's trying to deprive the viruses and bacteria of sugar, which is a ready food source for them. The body has a very sophisticated response to treat, with certain

(continued)

> ### *Expert Insight with Mr. Fintan Dunne (continued)*
>
> minerals etc. So help the fever along, the harsher the fever, within limits, the better it is for you. You can also take other things, like turmeric, ginger, or garlic — which contains selenium, onions, and fresh fruits and vegetables with a low sugar content (not oranges and bananas, which are high in sugar), meat for protein — that's an anti-influenza diet.
>
> **RK:** How high can you go with a fever and still be safe?
> **FD:** We tend to be a bit oversensitive about the issue of fever, and individual variations. You can certainly go to 104°F (40°C) without calling the paramedics. Febrile seizure is a concern, but it does have to be monitored, but we should not let our concern over what might happen in a small minority of individuals completely drive us away from fever, the body's optimal solution. And, febrile seizure — short-term febrile seizure is not a health threat, there's no evidence, there's no downside. We're way too sensitive to that, fever is our best friend, it is the body's natural response and we should just be going with that. There's good indications, for example in SARS, the people who got it were by and large the medical professionals who had quick and easy access to the widest range of drugs to mess around with the body's response. I'd almost rest my case on that.
>
> **RK:** Now, it is true that viruses are inhibited above temperature of 100°F (37.8°C).
> **FD:** Yes but there are any things responding he is doing as well. The immune system itself functions at its best at higher temperatures. So it is both inhibiting the virus and enhancing the immune response itself. … So I would say go with the body, when you get something. But it would be better not to get it in the first place.
>
> *Visit www.worldhealth.net/pandemic to listen to the entire interview with Mr. Dunne*

Treatment Protocol

There are three basic types of hyperthermia. Heating just a small portion of the body is called local hyperthermia and is sometimes used to treat upper respiratory infections or wounds. Regional hyperthermia refers to heating a larger area such as an arm or a leg. Whole-body hyperthermia is used as a cancer treatment. The heat selectively kills heat-sensitive malignancies. High-tech hyperthermia therapies involving application of electromagnetic energy, high-energy sound waves, infrared heat, or removing blood, heating it and returning it to the body must be done under the direction of an experienced healthcare practitioner.

Hot water bottles and baths, saunas and steam baths are less complicated forms of hyperthermia treatment you can prescribe for yourself for acute and chronic viral infections and chronic fatigue syndrome – as long as you do not abuse them. In 1989, a German study found that people who enjoyed saunas twice a week got half as many colds as those who did not (the suspected reason is the inhalation of air hotter than 80°F [26.7°C] – too hot for colds and flu viruses to survive and flourish). In addition, when your body temperature is slightly elevated due to an infection, consider skipping the aspirin, acetaminophen, ibuprofen, and any other fever-lowering medications, thus giving your body an opportunity to use the fever for its natural purpose – to kill or reduce the numbers of invading viruses and bacteria and to sweat pathogens out of the body. Temperatures over 104°F (40°C), however, call for immediate medical attention.

A number of strategies can be employed to break a fever. The easiest option is to take an antipyretic drug (a drug that lowers body temperature), such as acetaminophen or aspirin (note: aspirin should not be given to anyone under the age of 20), as they will help to reduce the fever. Another strategy is to bathe in tepid (not cold) water. Herbs that are diaphoretic (promote perspiration), such as chamomile, fennel, linden, and willow bark, will help break a fever, by increasing elimination of excess heat via the skin through perspiration. Herbs should be brewed as a tea (1 teaspoon of the mixture in 1 cup of boiling water for 5 minutes) and drunk several times a day.

Side Effect/Contraindications

People who have anemia, heart disease, diabetes, seizure disorders or tuberculosis should be extremely careful when using hyperthermia therapy, as should pregnant women. The very old and the very young, who may have trouble regulating body temperature, should avoid hyperthermia unless under a physician's close supervision.

Warning

Hyperthermia therapy is not without risk and can prove fatal. Adults should see a doctor right away if:

- Fever is 103°F (39.4°C) or higher
- Fever is prolonged
- Fever is accompanied by recurrent shaking or chills
- There are no apparent symptoms except a temperature of 101°F+ (38.3°C+) that lasts for more than 3 days
- There are no apparent symptoms except a low-grade fever lasting several weeks
- There has been known exposure to an infectious disease
- Fever is accompanied by severe headache, stiff neck, swelling of throat, or confusion/disorientation.

Consult your physician when treating fever, especially in children.

HYDROGEN PEROXIDE

Hydrogen peroxide is known to most people as a topical antiseptic or as an ingredient in mouthwash and toothpaste. It is composed of two hydrogen atoms and two oxygen atoms (H_2O_2). Proponents of H_2O_2 therapy believe it can be used in baths, nasal sprays, douches, colonics, and enemas. Binyamin Rothstein, D.O., an Osteopathic physician, gives his patients a very dilute concentration of hydrogen peroxide intravenously over a 90-minute to 3-hour period. "This therapy must be done carefully because it introduces very potent free radicals into the body," Rothstein explains. "Done the right way, it stimulates powerful antioxidant reactions. Hydrogen peroxide therapy is especially helpful in treating chronic and acute bronchitis, emphysema, sinusitis and chronic fatigue syndrome." Anecdotal reports suggest that it may also be useful for the treatment of influenza.

Treatment Protocol

Hydrogen peroxide can be used at home by adding a teaspoon of 3% hydrogen peroxide (H_2O_2), which can be bought at any pharmacy, to a glass of water. Alternatively, some sources recommend holding two teaspoons of hydrogen peroxide in the mouth for approximately three minutes, spitting it out, and then drinking a glass of water. However, it is also best to consult a qualified and experienced professional. For the treatment of flu take hydrogen peroxide as described above every hour from the onset of symptoms until you recover from the infection. Some sources recommend alternating the hydrogen peroxide with supplements like grape seed extract.

Side Effects/Contraindications

IMPORTANT: Do not use reagent-grade (35%) hydrogen peroxide internally, in any concentration.

Drinking water with 3% hydrogen peroxide can cause nausea. Hydrogen peroxide should be used with care. It should not be used on a daily basis as a general preventative as it will kill off the "good" bacteria in the gastrointestinal system.

RELAXATION

If you can teach yourself to relax, you can activate your immune system on demand. Formally known as psychoneuroimmunology, this is an active field of scientific research that studies the interaction among and between behaviors and emotions, the brain, and the immune system. The field of psychoneuroimmunology stems from healing traditions that are both ancient and modem, Eastern and Western.

One now famous study tested medical students during examination time. Their NK activity was reduced during exam time but returned to normal after exams. In another study, animals were injected with tumor cells. Those animals subjected to shocks over which they had no control developed tumors which grew more rapidly and death occurred more quickly. Those rats that were able to control the shock grew tumors at a lesser rate. Other studies have shown that relaxation triggers levels of interleukins -- leaders in the immune system response against cold and flu viruses -- in the bloodstream to rise.

Further studies, using the UCLA Loneliness Scale, have shown that people with higher loneliness scores had lower NK cell activity. Interestingly, in European studies it was found that depleting life events (such as divorce, loss of spouse, unemployment, loneliness) were not sole predictors for disease; rather, the particular coping style of the person seemed to be a predictor of development of disease.

Simply turn off all external stimulation (the radio, television, computer, phone, fax, etc) and sit quietly in a room, reflecting on pleasant thoughts, for 30 minutes every day. Relaxation is an active, learnable skill. It is not simply sitting and doing nothing. People who try to relax, but are in fact bored, show no changes in blood chemicals.

UV BLOOD IRRIDATION

UV blood irradiation (photopheresis or extracorporeal photochemotherapy) is a technique that has been in use since the 1930s when it was administered to thousands as a reliable and effective method to treat polio and sepsis. Lately, it has been making a comeback. The therapy involves placing a small amount of blood into a UV machine where a special wavelength of ultra-violet light kills viruses and bacteria. The treated blood is then reintroduced into the body. Ultra-violet blood irradiation introduces ultra-violet energy into the bloodstream, which is thought to produce small amounts of ozone from the oxygen circulating in the blood. Proponents of UV therapy claim it can destroy/inhibit the growth of bacteria, enhance the immune system's ability to fight infection, and successfully treat conditions such as viral infection, pneumonia, wound infections, septicemia, inflammatory processes (pancreatitis, bursitis, etc.), autoimmune diseases, immune deficiencies, and peripheral vascular disease. UV blood irradiation is an FDA-approved treatment for cutaneous T-cell lymphoma (a type of cancer affecting the skin.) Some evidence suggests that UV blood irradiation may prove useful in the treatment of immune system diseases, such as multiple sclerosis, rheumatoid arthritis, type I diabetes, systemic lupus erythematosus (SLE), and rejection of transplanted organs, and graft-versus-host disease.

Treatment Protocol

UV Blood irradiation is carried out under the direction of an experienced healthcare practitioner. During this procedure, blood is removed from the patient and separated into different types of cells. Approximately a pint of blood, which consists of mostly white blood cells, is treated with a drug to make it make it more sensitive to light. The blood is then treated with UV light, which activates the drug, and the blood is infused back into the patient. This procedure takes from 3 to 5 hours.

Side Effects/Contraindications

No significant side effects are associated with UV blood irradiation.

Natural Non-Drug Viral Inhibition

Viruses can be inhibited naturally by employing the following tactics:

- Maintain a body temperature of 101-102°F (38.3-38.8°C) (carefully read the section on "Fever" in the "Immunity Desk Reference" earlier in this chapter)
- Keep well hydrated (see Strategy #3, below): Drink 1 8-ounce (236 mL) glass of distilled water, with a pinch of salt (for electrolytes), every 1 to 2 hours that you are awake.
- Do deep breathing exercises (to expand your lungs and clear secretions from them) for 10 minutes, every 2 hours
- Take the key anti-viral nutrients, including (see individual entries in the "Immunity Desk Reference" earlier in this chapter):
  - Vitamin C: For the treatment of influenza, a daily dose of 1,000–6,000 mg is recommended
  - Selenium: 100-200mcg daily
  - Garlic: To fight infection, 3 or 4 chopped, crushed or chewed cloves should be consumed per day or, in supplement form (1.3% allicin), 600–900 mg divided into 2–3 doses/day
- Get some sunshine: 10-15 minutes of whole-body exposure to peak summer sun will generate and release up to 20,000 IU vitamin D, a potent immune system modulator, into circulation

---

Strategy #3. Hydration

Water is a nutrient essential to life. Humans can go days, even weeks, without food. Deprived of water, life can end within three days. Water composes more than half our bodies, one-quarter of our bones, and one-third of our brains. Water is present in every cell and tissue of the body and facilitates every bodily function, including respiration, digestion. cognition, and yes — immunity. Taking steps to make certain the quality of the water you consume is "grade A" is one of the most inexpensive yet most critical ways you can boost your resistance to infectious disease.

For many Americans, tap water exceeds the legal limits for dangerous contaminants such as parasites, bacteria and chemicals. New agricultural and industrial toxins are being introduced to the water supply at an alarming rate. In addition, scientists have identified bacteria usually found only in human feces in deep ocean waters, the result of human sewage disposal. That some of these bacteria are resistant to antibiotics is a clear sign that they originated in humans who were taking the drugs. In an ocean upwelling, these dormant pathogens can be brought to the surface—sometimes miles from their original dumping site.

Each year, as many as seven million people suffer gastrointestinal effects from drinking water (an especially dangerous threat for the very young and very old and for people with compromised immune systems). And in some places, experts speculate that contaminated water may cause birth defects, miscarriages and cancer.

The three most common water contaminants are cryptosporidium, lead and chlorine.

> Cryptosporidium. This parasite from animal fecal matter can cause even people with strong immune systems to suffer severe diarrhea and vomiting. In 1993, cryptosporidium contaminated the Milwaukee city water supply, sickening more than 400,000 people and killing 70. In 1998, children playing in a public fountain at a Minnesota zoo were infected. The source of the contamination may have been a child in diapers who played in the fountain.   Even though the fountain water was recirculated through a sand filter and then chlorinated, the pathogen survived.

> Lead. Millions of Americans are exposed to water that violates the EPA's 15 parts per billion limit. Excessive exposure to lead can cause high blood pressure, anemia, kidney damage and mental retardation. The most common sources of lead in drinking water are the lead pipes and solders commonly used before 1982.

> Chlorine. Since the early 1900s, chlorine has been used by water-treatment plants to kill disease-causing bacteria. Chlorine itself poses few direct health risks, but chlorine reacts with organic material in water to produce cancer-causing byproducts. It can also react with acids in water to form trihalomethanes (THMs), which have been linked to miscarriage and various cancers.

Don't Tap the Tap

In the U.S., 53 million Americans drink water from municipal water supplies containing potentially dangerous levels of chloro- and fluoro-chemicals, lead, fecal bacteria, as well as pesticides and other impurities associated with cancer and metabolic dysfunction.

Bottled and filtered water are better than tap water. Consider installing a water filtration system in your home, particularly for drinking and cooking needs. To make the most appropriate selection (based on contaminants present, daily use volume, and convenience), ask for recommendations from your plumber or local water department.

Inhaling steam vapors containing toxic metals is just as detrimental as consuming them. Consider installing a whole-house filtration system that purifies water supplying your bathrooms.

Opt for distilled, sterile water, which has the maximum ability to eliminate toxins from your body and is devoid of other substances and minerals. Add a pinch of salt, for electrolytes. If you drink *only* sterile distilled water, however, you lose not only toxic (heavy) metals by excretion through urine, but some of the beneficial minerals as well. Balance your diet with five or more servings of fruits and vegetables a day, and add a quality daily multimineral dietary supplement.

Tips for Healthy Hydration

<u>Stay alert to the quality of your water supply.</u>

The CDC reports that 900 deaths and one million cases of intestinal malaise each year are attributable to water-borne organisms.

The Environmental Working Group reports that 14 million people drink water contaminated with five of the most toxic herbicides. By doing so, 3.5 million people in our largest cities are at a cancer risk 10 times greater than the general population.

Most municipalities chlorinate water to kill dangerous microbes. Chlorine by-products thus wind up in the water supply of 100 million people, causing about 10,000 incidences of bladder cancer each year.

<u>First thing in the morning, run the cold water for at least 30 seconds</u> before ingesting, cooking, or offering a bowl to your pet. Many home plumbing systems are copper-based, and the minerals normally present in water may cause copper to leach from pipes as it sits overnight.

<u>Ask your local water department to provide you with a copy of the most recent analysis</u> of your water supply. Discuss your concerns relating to pesticides, radioactivity, and industrial wastes with the water department management or your town officials.

(continued)

Tips for Healthy Hydration *(continued)*

<u>Contact the bottler of your bottled water product</u> to ask for a copy of a complete independent analysis. There are over 450 bottling facilities in the U.S. producing more than 700 different brand labels of bottled water, creating a $2.2 billion industry (1990 estimates). Unsubstantiated health claims about bottled water are unlawful. All bottled water must come from a government-approved source, which must be inspected and the water sampled, analyzed, and found safe and sanitary with or without treatment. For additional bottled water information, contact the International Bottled Water Association (Alexandria, Virginia).

The best way to monitor fluid intake is to watch the color of your urine, which should be light rather than dark. Half of all the fluids you drink should be water. Tea, coffee, milk and juice count as fluids, but the water in foods (for example, fruits, vegetables and soups) does not. Consider that fluid a bonus. General guidelines for optimal fluid intake include:

- Aim for at least eight cups of fluid a day, half of them water.
  - Drink 1 8-ounce (236 mL) glass of distilled water, with a pinch of salt (for electrolytes), every 1 to 2 hours that you are awake. You may need to drink more when you are physically active.
- Drink some water first thing in the morning to make up for loss of fluids during the night.
- Drink a beverage with every meal.
- Don't wait until you are thirsty; drink throughout the day.
- For every cup of caffeinated beverage you drink, consume an extra half cup of another fluid to make up for caffeine's diuretic effect.

Some nutrition experts recommend daily water intake sufficient for detoxification to be 0.5 ounces (15 mL) per day per pound (0.45 kilogram) of body weight (which equates to 90 ounces [2.7 liters] per day for a 180-pound [82 kilogram] man). In times of metabolic stress (such as fighting an infection), intake should be increased by two- to three-fold.

Emergency Water Disinfection

In the event of a natural disaster, which may compromise your access to water from your tap or bottle source, follow these techniques to purify water for drinking:

- Boiling – vigorously, for 10 minutes
- Bleaching – add 10-20 drops of household bleach per gallon of water, mix well, and let stand for 30 minutes. A slight smell or taste of chlorine indicates water is good to drink. (Note: do not use scented bleaches, colorsafe bleaches, or bleaches with added cleaners.)
- Tablets – commercially available purification tablets
- Solar disinfection, known as SODIS — a new technique developed by researchers at the Swiss Federal Institute for Environmental Science and Technology in Duebendorf in which clear plastic bottles are filled with water and left in the sun. The heat warms the water and the combination of warm water and ultraviolet radiation kills most microorganisms. The Institute's tests showed that 99.9% of the E. coli in a sample of contaminated water were killed when the sun heated the water beyond 122°F (50°C). At that temperature, disinfection takes about an hour, but placing a corrugated metal sheet under the bottle can shorten the time. Additional tests demonstrate SODIS as an effective approach for killing the cholera bacteria, Vibrio cholerae, and that it could inactivate parasites including the diarrhea-causing Cryptosporidium. The Institute is widely promoting SODIS in Asia and South America.

Strategy #4. Daily Nutrition

Individuals should aim to eat a balanced diet every day, consisting of a variety of foods, to help maintain physical strength and promote optimal immune function:

- Consume 3 ounces (0.085 kilograms) or more, every day, of whole grain foods (bread, cereal, crackers, rice, pasta)
- Additionally, aim for 2-3 cups (0.45-0.68 kilograms) of vegetables and 2 cups (0.45 kilograms) of fruit each day. Choose vibrantly colored — dark green, red, and yellow — fruits and vegetables, which tend to have higher concentrations of immune-enhancing phytochemicals.
- Enhance your meals with lean or low-fat sources of protein: 5-6 ounces (0.14-0.17 kilograms) per day of meats, poultry, fish, dry beans/peas, eggs, nuts, and/or seeds
- Enjoy 3 cups (0.68 kg) per day of low-fat or fat-free milk, cheese, or yogurt
- Avoid: processed or preserved foods; foods that are rich in fat, cholesterol, salt and sugar

For personalized meal plans and tips, log on to the U.S. Department of Agriculture's Food Pyramid website at http://www.mypyramid.gov.

Foods to Avoid If You Have the Flu

- Sugary foods: Sugars are the food on which viruses feast, so resist sweets to starve the pathogens making you sick.
- Bananas, oranges (and citrus juices), peanuts, and dairy: Avoid these foods that increase mucous formation, which enables an internal environment that is conducive to harboring viruses.

With the spread of H5N1 through Asia and Eastern Europe, fermented cabbage products are experiencing a soar in popularity. Kimchi is a Korean dish of pickled cabbage and spices. Rich in vitamins, kimchi has been shown to have anti-cancer activity, and during the SARS crisis of 2003 many Koreans believed eating kimchi helped ward off the disease.

Sauerkraut is the European counterpart to kimchi, made in a similar fermentation process. A 2005 study by Polish and American scientists have proposed that sauerkraut, contributes to the lower breast cancer rate observed among Polish immigrants in America. The food is rich in glucosinolates — compounds demonstrated to have anti-cancer activity in the lab. Glucosinolates are preserved in sauerkraut, as the compounds are destroyed when the cabbage is cooked.

In November 2005, Sa-ouk Kang and colleagues at Seoul National University (South Korea) reported that the lactic acid bacteria strain *Leuconostoc Kimchii* was able to help 11 of 13 chickens with bird flu recover from the disease. In a lab experiment testing the bacteria on bird flu in humans, Professor Kang reported a "very potent effect."

Spiced Air

In February 2006, South Korean firm LG Electronics announced it would start marketing in Asia an air conditioner with a filter made using an enzyme from kimchi. Because the filter is made with only the enzyme extracted from kimchi, the air conditioner does not emit the pungent aroma that characterizes the dish.

Strategy #5. Poultry Safety

On-going outbreaks of highly pathogenic H5N1 avian influenza in poultry in Asia and, more recently, in Europe and Africa have raised grave concerns about multiple sources of infection and the risk to humans from various exposures. The greatest risk of exposure to the virus is through the handling and slaughter of live infected poultry. Good hygiene practices are essential during slaughter and post- slaughter handling to prevent exposure via raw poultry meat or cross contamination from poultry to other foods, food preparation surfaces or equipment.

Most strains of avian influenza virus are found only in the respiratory and gastrointestinal tracts of infected birds, and not in meat. However, available studies indicate that highly pathogenic viruses, such as the H5N1 strain, spread to virtually all parts of an infected bird, including meat. <u>Avian influenza viruses survive in contaminated raw poultry meat and therefore can be spread through the marketing and distribution of contaminated food products, such as fresh or frozen meat.</u>

The U.S. government regulates domestic and imported food products, and in 2004 issued a ban on importation of poultry from countries affected by avian influenza viruses, including the H5N1 strain. This ban still is in place. As of 1 May 2006, bans by the U.S. Department of Agriculture (USDA) on the following countries due to the presence of the H5N1 strain of avian influenza in commercial flocks are in effect: Cambodia, Egypt, India, Indonesia, Japan, Laos, Kazakhstan, Malaysia, Nigeria, People's Republic of China, Romania, Russia, South Korea, Thailand, Turkey, Ukraine, and Vietnam. Processed poultry products from these countries must be accompanied by a USDA permit.

Most recently, on 25 February 2006, the USDA's Animal and Plant Health Inspection Service (APHIS) has placed a temporary ban on the importation of poultry and commercial shipments of live birds, hatching eggs and unprocessed avian products from the French Department (state) of Ain based on the diagnosis of highly pathogenic avian influenza H5N1 in commercially raised turkeys. The restriction is only on the Department of Ain, not the entire country of France. In addition, this ban provides that U.S.-origin pet birds and performing birds will be allowed to return from France only after entering one of the three USDA Quarantine Centers for 30 days.

Facts About H5N1 in Poultry

- The H5N1 virus, if present in poultry meat, is not killed by refrigeration or freezing. In general, low temperatures maintain the viability of the avian influenza virus. The virus can survive in feces for at least 35 days at low temperature (39.2°F [4°C]); while at 98.6°F (37°C), viruses could survive for 6 days in stability tests on fecal samples in studies using H5N1 viruses circulating during 2004. (Feces may come into contact with poultry meat during the slaughtering process.)
- Eggs can contain H5N1 virus both on the outside (shell) and the inside (whites and yolk). Eggs from areas with H5N1 outbreaks in poultry should not be consumed raw or partially cooked (runny yolk); uncooked eggs should not be used in foods that will not be cooked, baked or heat-treated in other ways.
- There have been reports of a few human cases of H5N1 potentially linked to consumption of raw poultry ingredients (such as raw blood-based dishes). It should therefore be emphasized that consumption of any raw poultry ingredients must be considered a high-risk practice and discouraged. This message is important not only for avian influenza, but also for preventing a range of other diseases transmitted through raw or undercooked poultry (including salmonella).

The GI Tract as a Route of Transmission or First Infection

Virologist Menno de Jong from Oxford University Clinical Research Unit (Vietnam) has proposed that bird flu may be capable of invading people thorough the gut, not just the respiratory system. He suggests that particles of the H5N1 virus contained in the meat and blood of infected poultry may be ingested to cause infection. He cites the Asian custom of drinking raw duck blood, which has made a number of people sick with H5N1. According to Dr. de Jong, this could imply that <u>the gastrointestinal tract is also a route of transmission — or route of first infection.</u>

Warns Dr. de Jong: If live virus particles are carried outside the lungs and surrounding tissues to other parts of the body, <u>inhaled antiviral treatments (such as zanamivir [Relenza]) may not be effective.</u> (See Chapter 4.)

The World Health Organization (WHO) reports that no epidemiological data suggest that the disease can be transmitted to humans through properly cooked food (even if contaminated with the virus prior to cooking). U.S. government officials at the HHS Department also agree that there is no evidence that properly cooked poultry or eggs can be a source of infection for avian influenza viruses. Cooking kills the H5N1 virus extremely quickly (within seconds of reaching 158°F [70°C]). In addition, proper food handling — including that of raw chicken and eggs — is crucial.

Food Handling Tips
"Five Keys to Safer Food," Issued by The World Health Organization

In 2001 the WHO introduced the Five Keys, simple rules elaborated to promote safer food handling and preparation practices. According to WHO, following the Five Keys not only prevents illness from eating contaminated food but also contributes to the prevention of diseases caused by handling infected animals, such as avian influenza.

<u>Key 1. Keep clean</u>
- Wash your hands before handling food and often during food preparation
- Wash your hands after going to the toilet
- Wash and sanitize all surfaces and equipment used for food preparation
- Protect kitchen areas and food from insects, pests and other animals

<u>Key 2. Separate raw and cooked</u>
- Separate raw meat, poultry and seafood from other foods
- Use separate equipment and utensils such as knives and cutting boards for handling raw foods
- Store food in containers to avoid contact between raw and prepared foods

(continued)

Food Handling Tips *(continued)*

<u>Key 3. Cook thoroughly</u>
- Cook food thoroughly, especially meat, poultry, eggs and seafood
- Bring foods like soups and stews to boiling to make sure that they have reached 158°F (70°C). For meat and poultry, make sure that juices are clear, not pink. Ideally, use a thermometer.
- Reheat cooked food thoroughly

<u>Key 4. Keep food at safe temperatures</u>
- Do not leave cooked food at room temperature for more than 2 hours
- Refrigerate promptly all cooked and perishable food (preferably below 41°F [5°C])
- Keep cooked food piping hot (more than 140°F [60°C]) prior to serving
- Do not store food too long even in the refrigerator
- Do not thaw frozen food at room temperature

<u>Key 5. Use safe water and raw materials</u>
- Use safe (potable) water or treat it to make it safe
- Select fresh and wholesome foods
- Choose foods processed for safety, such as pasteurized milk and juices
- Wash fruits and vegetables, especially if eaten raw
- Do not use food beyond its expiry date

Checklist for Safe Poultry Preparation
Issued by The World Health Organization's International Food Safety Authorities Network (INFOSAN)
- <u>Separate raw meat from cooked or ready-to-eat foods.</u> Do not use the same chopping board or the same knife for raw chicken and other foods. Do not handle both raw and cooked chicken without washing your hands in between and do not place cooked chicken back on the same plate or surface it was on before cooking. Do not use raw or soft-boiled eggs in food preparations that will not be heat treated or cooked.
- <u>Keep clean and wash your hands.</u> After handling frozen or thawed raw chicken or eggs, wash your hands thoroughly with soap. Wash and disinfect all surfaces and utensils that have been in contact with the raw meat.
- <u>Cook thoroughly.</u> Thorough cooking of poultry meat will inactivate the virus. Either ensure that the poultry meat reaches 158°F (70°C) at the center of the product ("piping" hot) or that the meat is not pink in any part. Egg yolks should not be runny or liquid.
- <u>Do not eat raw poultry parts or raw eggs.</u>

Additionally, soapy water and detergents are an important first-line defense against picking up and/or spreading the H5N1 virus. The avian influenza virus is more simple to destroy than many viruses since it is very sensitive to detergents which destroy the fat containing outer layer of the virus. This layer is needed to enter cells of animals and therefore destroying it destroys the viral infectivity. Therefore, frequent and thorough handwashing while preparing and serving food is critical (see Strategy #1 above).

Strategy #6. Face Masks & Respirators

According to the U.S. Implementation Plan for the National Strategy for Pandemic Influenza, released 3 May 2006: "The benefit of wearing disposable surgical or procedure masks at school or in the workplace has not been established. Mask use by the public should be based on risk, including the frequency of exposure and closeness of contact with potentially infectious persons. Routine mask use in public should be permitted, but not required."

The federal government urges that "during a pandemic, persons who are diagnosed with influenza or who have a febrile respiratory illness should remain at home until the fever is resolved and the cough is resolving to avoid exposing others. If such symptomatic persons cannot stay home during the acute phase of their illness, consideration should be given to having them wear a surgical or procedure mask in public places when they may have close contact with other persons."

Further, these guidelines state: "Although the use of surgical or procedure masks by asymptomatic individuals in community settings has not been demonstrated to be a public health measure to decrease infections during a community outbreak, persons may choose to wear a mask as part of individual protection strategies that include cough etiquette, hand hygiene, and avoiding public gatherings. If persons at risk for complications of influenza decide to wear masks during periods of increased respiratory illness activity in the community, it is likely they will need to wear them any time they are in a public place and when they are around other household members."

Both the World Health Organization (WHO) and the U.S. Centers for Disease Control & Prevention (CDC) recommend the use of personal protective equipment (PPE) to minimize direct contact with the influenza virus in at-risk populations. U.S. NIOSH certified N-95 disposable face masks are recognized as effective barriers for influenza. N95 disposable face masks have two advantages over simple cloth or surgical masks:

1. They are >95% efficient at filtering 0.3-μm particles (smaller than the 5-μm size of large droplets—created during talking, coughing, and sneezing—which usually transmit influenza);
2. They are fit-tested to ensure that infectious droplets and particles do not leak around the mask. Even if N95 filtration is unnecessary for avian influenza, N95 fit offers advantages over a loose-fitting surgical mask by eliminating leakage around the mask.

Mask Use Guidelines
- Wash hands before putting on a mask, and before and after taking one off.
- The mask should fit snugly over the face, fully covering the nose, mouth and chin.
- Try not to touch the mask once it is secured on your face as frequent handling may reduce its protection. If you must do so, wash your hands before and after touching the mask.
- When taking off the mask, avoid touching the outside of the mask as this part may be covered with germs.
- After taking off the mask, put the mask into a plastic or paper bag before putting it into a lidded rubbish bin.
- Change the mask at least daily. Replace the mask immediately if it is damaged or soiled.
- Any mask must be disposed of if it becomes moist.
- Do not share your mask with anyone else.
- To avoid physical deterioration of the mask during use, men should be clean-shaven (no mustache or beard).

Extending Mask Life – In the Condition of Emergency Shortages of Masks *ONLY*
As a general rule, do not reuse masks, as they can rapidly lose their protective function. However, in the event that masks become limited in supply and you have no option but to reuse a used mask, consider the following options:
- Insert a paper towel, cotton handkerchief, or piece of a cotton T-shirt, folded 2 or more times, inside your mask. Every 1 to 2 hours, replace the insert. This option attempts to keep moisture away from your mask, which can compromise its lifespan and efficacy.
- Dry and decontaminate used masks in an oven, set at 165°F (74°C) to 200°F (93.3°C), for 15 minutes, taking care not to burn the mask.

If, at any time, the texture feels or appears burned, brittle, or weakened, do not reuse the mask.

Strategy #7. Barriers

The influenza virus, including H5N1, transmits via the respiratory and mucosal tracts. As we discussed earlier (see "Personal Space Safety" in Strategy #1 above), a sneeze or cough can propel a virus 10 or more feet (3 or more meters). Human influenza virus can transmit from person-to-person across a distance of 3 feet (1 meter), and also may occur through direct and indirect contact with infectious respiratory secretions. So it is essential to protect the mouth, nose, and eyes from direct contact with the pathogen.

Face masks and respirators (see Strategy #6 above) may confer some protection for the mouth and nose. Because face masks do not cover your eyes — leaving them susceptible as a viral point of entry — you should also wear eyeglasses, sunglasses, or safety goggles. At all times, avoid rubbing your eyes with your hands. Most of all, proper hygiene (see Strategy #1 above) is absolutely critical.

Strategy #8. Ventilation

The H5N1 virus spreads through the air. At present, it can be transmitted from infected live birds to humans. Human-to-human transmission has not yet been documented.

People in close contact with poultry are more susceptible to contracting bird flu. The elderly, children, and people with chronic illness are specific subpopulations that, once contracting bird flu, may develop severe complications such bronchitis and pneumonia.

It is important to:

- Maintain good indoor ventilation, so as to minimize the lingering of virus particles in the air
- Avoid crowded places with poor ventilation if you are feeling unwell, so as not to risk contaminating others

Use a HEPA (high-efficiency particulate air) filter on your whole-house ventilation system, as these can serve as a barricade preventing the circulation of infectious particles.

There has been new interest in UV-C, or short-wave ultraviolet radiation, which attacks the DNA of a cell. This wavelength is utilized in certain ventilation systems in the healthcare setting to destroy viruses, bacteria, mold and other microorganisms. Influenza requires 3,400 microwatts of UV-C energy for complete destruction (10,000 microwatts are required to destroy tuberculosis). A number of hospitals worldwide are now considering installation of UV-C systems facility-wide in preparation for a possible pandemic. UV-C systems are available for homes, but can be very expensive to purchase and maintain.

Strategy #9. Humidification

Virus epidemics are far more prevalent during winter months. Possible reasons include:

1. Cold, dry air inhibits natural viral cleansing of respiratory passages and immobilizes cilia, the tiny hairs that move debris and germs out of the nasal passage and lungs
2. Dry air dehydrates respiratory passages, starting cracks and dents in the mucosa, making for easier delivery of viral infectious particles
3. Less sun exposure, which results with less natural production by the body of Vitamin D, a potent immune system modulator (see "Vitamin D" in the "Immunity Desk Reference" earlier in this chapter)

In the winter, wear a scarf to cover the mouth and nose, to prewarm and humidify the cold winter air before you breathe it in.

Strategy #10. Safe & Smart Travel

If you have a cough (as a result of any illness), you should be courteous to fellow travelers. Avoid infecting others by:

- Wearing a face mask (see Strategy #6 earlier in this chapter);
- Coughing into a paper towel several layers thick, and dispose of the towel right away; and
- Frequently and properly washing your hands (see Strategy #1 earlier in this chapter), and use an alcohol-based hand cleaner in-between handwashings.

Conversely, people should be wary of fellow travelers who have a cough (as a result of any illness). The same basic hygiene suggestions apply.

To improve air circulation during airplane travel, ask the flight crew to open the "air packs" that provide fresh air within the passenger cabin, and to turn off recirculation fans. It is standard operating procedure for pilots to turn off 30% of the air supply, since it costs more than $100 an hour for a 747 to run a single air pack. Frugality is commendable, but the money the airlines save could cost you and your fellow passengers your lives.

Travel to H5N1 Affected Areas

As of 1 May 2006, the U.S. Centers for Disease Control & Prevention has not recommended that the general public avoid travel to any of the countries affected by H5N1. For a current list of countries reporting outbreaks of H5N1 infection among poultry and other birds and a list of countries reporting laboratory-confirmed human infections with H5N1 viruses, see the CDC webpage at http://www.cdc.gov/flu/avian/outbreaks/current.htm.

Pandemic: Not a question of *"if,"* but *"when"* ...
English Clergyman Thomas Fuller (1608-1661) remarked: "In fair weather prepare for foul." A prudent individual will prepare for disaster before it is on the doorstep.

Log on to **www.worldhealth.net/pandemic** every week to read the latest tips for protecting yourself and your loved ones from the wrath of an impending infectious disease outbreak.

LEXMD.com
Physicians' picks of the "best of the best" of essential anti-aging health products that can help you live a long, healthy, vital, robust, and productive life. All products offered at **www.lexmd.com** are backed by a 100% absolute satisfaction, no-hassle, money-back guarantee. Read more information about natural immune-optimizing approaches at **www.lexmd.com**.

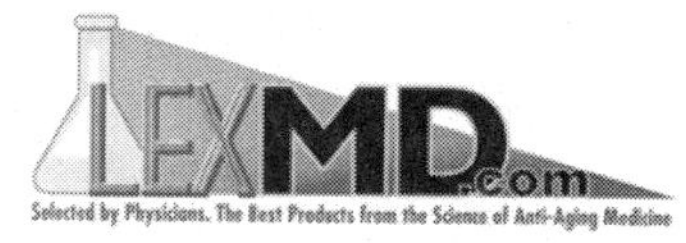

www.lexmd.com

The CDC recommendations for persons visiting areas with reports of outbreaks of H5N1 among poultry or of human H5N1 are as follows:

Before Any International Travel to An Area Affected by H5N1 Avian Influenza

- Visit CDC's Travelers' Health website at http://www.cdc.gov/travel to educate yourself and others who may be traveling with you about any disease risks and CDC health recommendations for international travel in areas you plan to visit.
- Be sure you are up to date with all your routine vaccinations, and see your doctor or health-care provider, ideally 4–6 weeks before travel, to get any additional vaccination medications or information you may need.
- Assemble a travel health kit containing basic first aid and medical supplies. Be sure to include a thermometer and alcohol-based hand gel for hand hygiene. See the Travelers Health Kit page in Health Information for International Travel (http://www2.ncid.cdc.gov/travel/yb/utils/ybGet.asp?section=recs&obj=travelers-health-kit.htm) for other suggested items.
- Identify in-country health-care resources in advance of your trip.
- Check your health insurance plan or get additional insurance that covers medical evacuation in case you become sick. Information about medical evacuation services is provided on the U.S. Department of State webpage on Medical Information for Americans Traveling Abroad, at http://travel.state.gov/travel/tips/health/health_1185.html.

During Travel to An Affected Area

- Avoid all direct contact with poultry, including touching well-appearing, sick, or dead chickens and ducks. Avoid places such as poultry farms and bird markets where live poultry are raised or kept, and avoid handling surfaces contaminated with poultry feces or secretions.
- As with other infectious illnesses, one of the most important preventive practices is careful and frequent handwashing (see Strategy #1 earlier in this chapter). Cleaning your hands often with soap and water removes potentially infectious material from your skin and helps prevent disease transmission. Waterless alcohol-based hand gels may be used when soap is not available and hands are not visibly soiled.
- All foods from poultry, including eggs and poultry blood should be cooked thoroughly. Egg yolks should not be runny or liquid. Because influenza viruses are destroyed by heat, the cooking temperature for poultry meat should be 165°F (74°C).
- If you become sick with symptoms such as a fever accompanied by a cough, sore throat, or difficulty breathing or if you develop any illness that requires prompt medical attention, a U.S. consular officer can assist you in locating medical services and informing your family or friends. Inform your health-care provider of any possible

(continued)

During Travel to An Affected Area *(continued)*

exposures to avian influenza. See Seeking Health Care Abroad in Health Information for International Travel (http://www2.ncid.cdc.gov/travel/yb/utils/ybGet.asp?section=recs&obj=care-abroad.htm) for more information about what to do if you become ill while abroad. You should defer further travel until you are free of symptoms, unless traveling locally for medical care.

Note: Some countries have instituted health monitoring techniques, such as temperature screenings, at ports of entry of travelers arriving from areas affected by avian influenza. Please consult the Embassy of your travel destination country if you have any questions.

After Your Return
- Monitor your health for 10 days.
- If you become ill with a fever plus a cough, sore throat, or trouble breathing during this 10-day period, consult a health-care provider. Before you visit a health-care setting, tell the provider the following: 1) your symptoms, 2) where you traveled, and 3) if you have had direct contact with poultry or close contact with a severely ill person. This way, he or she can be aware that you have traveled to an area reporting avian influenza.
- Do not travel while ill, unless you are seeking medical care. Limiting contact with others as much as possible can help prevent the spread of an infectious illness.

Chapter 4. Bird Flu Treatment Options

Historically Successful Interventions for Pandemic Flu

During the 1918 flu pandemic, osteopathic (D.O.) medical hospitals treated flu and pneumonia victims with therapies including Osteopathic Manipulative Treatment (OMT), lymphatic pump, postural drainage, and hydration. The death rate among this group was just 0.25%, whereas patients treated at allopathic (M.D.) hospitals stood at 6%. Osteopathic treatment of influenza-related pneumonia resulted with a 10% death rate, whereas M.D.-administered treatment yielded a 33 to 75% death rate on-average. Additionally, chiropractors caring for influenza patients during the 1918 flu pandemic lost far fewer patients than M.D.s; similarly, it is also reported that homeopaths lost only 5-6% of their flu patients.

The commonality between osteopathic, chiropractic, and homeopathic treatment of flu patients during the 1918 pandemic is that they relied solely on natural, non-toxic, non-pharmacological interventive approaches.

Osteopathic Manipulative Treatment (OMT)

Osteopathic manipulative treatment, or OMT, is hands-on care. It involves using the hands to diagnose, treat, and prevent illness or injury. Using OMT, your osteopathic physician (D.O.) will move your muscles and joints using techniques including stretching, gentle pressure and resistance. OMT can help people of all ages and backgrounds, serving to ease pain, promote healing, and increase mobility. Often, OMT is used to treat muscle pain, and can also help patients with a number of other health problems, including asthma, sinus disorder, carpal tunnel syndrome, migraines, and menstrual pain. When medically appropriate, OMT can complement—and even replace—drugs or surgery. In this way, OMT brings an important dimension to standard medical care.

OMT is of particular benefit to treat the symptoms of influenza, because it can help break up mucous secretions and mitigate the sympathetic connection between the spinal cord and lungs. As shown during the 1918 flu pandemic, OMT techniques can be lifesaving. In 1918, the most effective osteopathic treatment during the influenza pandemic was begun early in the onset of symptoms (within the first 24 hours), and consisted of carefully applied muscle relaxation, and most importantly, relaxation of the deep and extensive contractions of the deep spinal musculature and mobilization of the spine. These treatments were repeated 2 to 6 times per day, early in the course of infection. During the later phases of infection, OMT likely enhanced lymphatic drainage and modulated an overactive immune response that exacerbated the condition by causing unwanted systemic inflammation. OMT was historically successful in treating pandemic flu because of a strong emphasis on mobilizing airway secretions, and prevention of rib and spinal muscle spasms that limit respiration. In addition, it is believed that deep tissue massage provided by OMT modulated sympathetic system tone, helping to keep airways open.

Chest Percussion

Chest percussion is a western adaptation of the Hitting Method of the Tao System of Traditional Chinese Medicine. Vibrations that are created and deliberate can effectively break up thick secretions commonly associated with respiratory infections. With a firm but gentle strike of the palm side of a cupped hand, the practitioner will move along the center of the upper rib cage downward until the bottom of the rib cage, tapping 10 to 12 times every 4 or so inches apart. The cupping delivers a maximal vibration that penetrates the chest cavity, bronchial tree, and the depths of the lungs, loosening thick mucous secretions. The action of the cilia (tiny hairs that direct the flow of air and sputum) will clear the loosened mucus and restore your fuller breathing capacity.

Similar rapid but low intensity cupping over the sternum is useful in stimulating the thymus, an important organ of immunity.

IMPORTANT: Do not use chest percussion if you: are experiencing chest pain; have fractured ribs; are experiencing an irregular pulse; or have a tendency to bleed (or are taking any blood thinners).

Lymphatic Pump

The immunologic response to infection or vaccine is generated in the lymph nodes. Lymphatic fluid from tissue or from an injection site is channeled by the lymphatic vessels to the lymph nodes where T-cells and B cells are activated. The lymphatic pump is a manipulative technique developed by Osteopathic physicians and performed by D.O.s and trained health professionals. The objective is to facilitate the movement through the body's natural filtration system by stimulating the movement of lymphatic fluid. It has proven to be remarkably effective at stimulating immunity and helping to reduce the discomfort of any condition in which thick mucous build-up hinders clear breathing.

During the later influenza epidemics (such as the 1928-1929 and 1936-1937 outbreaks), lymphatic pump treatment, along with more attention to the cervical and upper thoracic regions, were added to the original 1918 osteopathic protocol (see "Osteopathic Manipulative Treatment" above). These treatments could be individualized to each patient's needs and were among the most commonly applied osteopathic medical procedures during past flu epidemics.

Therapeutic Massage

Research suggests that medical massage can strengthen the immune system, relieve pain, reduce damaging stress hormones, and alleviate symptoms of depression and anxiety. Massage also has been linked to reducing inflammation, helping people with asthma breathe easier, alleviate chronic fatigue and migraines, and ease the symptoms of irritable bowel syndrome. Scientists speculate that massage accomplishes all this by improving circulation, boosting the flow of lymph, flushing out lactic acid and stimulating the release of endorphins.

Homeopathy

Based on the principle that 'like cures like,' the word 'homeopathy' is a combination of Greek words meaning 'similar disease.' Samuel Hahnemann, a German physician practicing in the late 1700s. developed a theory based on the three principles that subsequently formed the foundation of the homeopathic tradition: (1) the law of similars; (2) the minimum dose; and (3) the single remedy. It is an approach that treats disease by administering minute, vanishingly small, highly diluted quantities of an agent (typically on the order of 10^{-6} to 10^{-10} and beyond), on the premise that such dosing will that evoke the same symptoms in the ill person (to build tolerance) as the disease when given to a healthy individual.

Homeopathy is often compared to antigen sensitivity as administered by an allergist or vaccinologist, where the tiniest amounts of antigen can promote system-wide beneficial effects. Some homeopathic remedies are so dilute that no molecules of the proposed healing substance remain; instead, homeopathic practitioners believe the substance has left its "imprint," or molecular memory, on the solution, that enables stimulation of the cells of the body.

It is strongly recommended that those seeking a homeopathic practitioner first check the status of their practitioner's State licensing.

Medications

Antiviral drugs are medicines given to people either prophylactically to prevent influenza or therapeutically once they are already infected.

Four different influenza antiviral drugs (amantadine, rimantadine, oseltamivir, and zanamivir) are approved by the U.S. Food and Drug Administration (FDA) for the treatment and prevention of influenza.

Genetic sequencing of the H5N1 virus from human cases in Vietnam and Thailand shows that the circulating H5N1 influenza virus is resistant to the two older (and less expensive) antiviral drugs, rimantadine and amantadine. Scientists are studying how the H5N1 viruses became resistant to these older drugs and carefully watching for any signs of resistance to the newer drugs.

Data from the World Health Organization's Global Influenza Surveillance Network indicate that the recently circulating H5N1 strains are susceptible to two antiviral drugs approved for use in the United States to treat human influenza infections – oseltamivir (sold as Tamiflu) and zanamivir (sold as Relenza). However, these medicines need to be started early enough – usually within the first two days of infection – to be effective. Some experts suggest Tamiflu needs to be given propholactically to work.

A New Mechanism of Action

Both oseltamivir (Tamiflu) and zanamivir (Relenza) belong to a new class of antiviral drugs called *neuraminidase inhibitors*. The surfaces of influenza viruses are dotted with neuraminidase proteins (see "Bird's Eye View of Bird Flu" in Chapter 2). Neuraminidase, an enzyme, breaks the bonds that hold new virus particles to the outside of an infected cell. Once the enzyme breaks these bonds, this sets free new viruses that can infect other cells and spread infection. Neuraminidase inhibitors block the enzyme's activity and prevent new virus particles from being released, thereby limiting the spread of infection.

Many experts say that for containment of H5N1 to be successful, the window of opportunity is on the order of "two to three weeks after signs of a pandemic emerge. If we fail, the consequences for societies, economies, and global public health could be immeasurable," remarks Japanese Deputy Foreign Minister Mitoshi Yabunaka.

Oseltamivir

Oseltamivir (Tamiflu) is an oral anti-viral medicine. The active ingredient, shikimic acid, is extracted from star anise, a spice grown mostly in China. Tamiflu also contains compounds derived from fermented E. coli bacteria.

Tamiflu does not prevent the individual from being infected by the virus, it prevents replication of the virus from already infected cells. Tamiflu treats some types of influenza in patients who have had symptoms of the flu for 2 days or less. Tamiflu also helps shorten the time a person has flu symptoms.

To treat influenza in adults, Tamiflu is dosed at 75 mg twice-daily for five days, beginning within 2 days of the appearance of symptoms. However, to treat H5N1 infection, higher doses and longer duration of therapy have been recommended. Scientists have warned that if the dose of Tamiflu is insufficient to treat the virus, resistance to the medicine may develop and render the medicine ineffective.

When taken as directed to prevent the flu, Tamiflu can significantly reduce an individual's chance of getting Influenza A if there is a flu outbreak in a family or community. Because H5N1 is a strain of Influenza A, popular opinion presumes that Tamiflu will also act as an effective prophylactic against bird flu. However, medical experts expect Tamiflu to be the most useful in helping to contain a pandemic in its early stages as a localized outbreak, and is not considered as a primary weapon in the fight against bird flu pandemic.

Problems with Prophylactic Tamiflu

<u>Problem #1.</u> Prophylactic Tamiflu must be given continuously during the entire length of an outbreak in order to remain effective. That amounts to an astronomical requirement of Tamiflu to protect the entire world population

<u>Problem #2.</u> Tamiflu has not been tested for long-term safety and efficacy in humans. It has been taken safely by large at-risk groups such as nursing home residents for periods of several weeks at a time, only.

<u>Problem #3.</u> Its usage by non-medical personnel, including civilians, is not prudent because issues as simple as its handling and transport may negate its desired effects. Tamiflu needs to be stored at room temperature between 59 to 77 °F (15-25°C) to avoid spoilage. Exposure to high temperature during shipping may render it useless.

The World Health Network
www.worldhealth.net
Serving over 20 million hits a month
Established in 1996

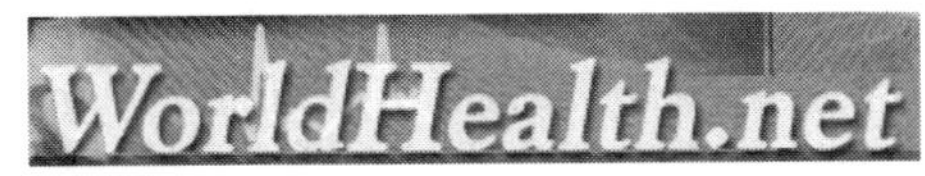

The #1 respected source of scientific and referenced clinical information on all issues of personal health, fitness, nutritional medicine, biomedical technologies, and anti-aging medicine —for immune health and overall longevity.

The Tamiflu Shortage

The World Health Organization suggested that every country should stockpile enough Tamiflu to treat at least a quarter of their population, amounting to a minimum of 20 billion doses.

Tamiflu is made nearly exclusively by the Swiss firm, Roche, which estimates producing 400 million courses of treatment by the end of 2006. But even then, it will take years to produce the emergency stockpiles that countries around the world have ordered.

At present, Tamiflu manufacturing is a slow process, involving ten individual steps that take over a year to complete. Tamiflu manufacture requires sodium azide, a highly explosive chemical. As a result, Tamiflu can be made only in small batches of a few tens of liters at a time. However, a Harvard University researcher has devised a new way to make Tamiflu without the inclusion of azide, which is hoped to allow continuous production — versus batch production — in the near future.

Large-scale Tamiflu production is also hindered by the fact that the patent on Tamiflu does not expire in 2016. Until then, any company wishing to manufacture Tamiflu must do so by securing the permission of the patent holder, Roche. This can be an expensive endeavor.

The Tamiflu Stockpile

International stockpiles of Tamiflu presently amount to 3 million treatment courses, which are stored in Switzerland and the United States. As of May 2006, the Asian region — the epicenter of the H5N1 outbreak — did not have a Tamiflu stockpile, but is aiming to have 500,000 courses as part of the Association of Southeast Asian Nations (ASEAN) project to fight H5N1.

The exact dosing of Tamiflu for use in treating bird flu in humans remains undetermined. A study by a team from St. Jude's Children's Hospital (Memphis, Tennessee) and announced in May 2006, studied ferrets given Tamiflu after being infected with the H5N1 virus. It illustrated the benefits of early treatment and the results are in-line with the limited research available about using Tamiflu to fight H5N1 in humans. After being infected for 4 hours, ferrets were given a dose equal to half the conventional human dosage for 5 days, saving their lives. A higher dose was also given to a group of animals 24 hours after being infected; again, all the animals survived. In both instances, all the untreated animals died. This research is now being used to predict how much Tamiflu people will need to take and for how long, to fight an H5N1 infection.

Side effects of Tamiflu include nausea, vomiting, bronchitis, difficulty sleeping, and dizziness.

Zanamivir

Zanamivir (Relenza) is a powdered medicine that is inhaled using a specially designed apparatus. As an inhaleable powder, it is of limited usefulness in asthmatics and people with respiratory difficulties.

For treatment of Influenza A, the recommended dosage is two inhalations twice a day, morning and night, for 5 days. Relenza is not currently considered a viable prophylactic treatment.

Headache and diarrhea are the most common side effects of Relenza.

U.S. Stockpile of Antivirals Insufficient

A study published in the 28 April 2006 issue of the scientific journal *Nature* (Volume 440 Number 7088, pgs. 1089-1244) recommending the rapid treatment of infected people and quarantine of entire households to reduce the disease rates by 50% warns that the strategy requires antiviral stockpiles sufficient to treat 50% of the population. Presently, the U.S. has enough antiviral drugs to treat 1% of the nation's population. The Department of Health & Human Services (HHS) plans to stockpile antivirals sufficient to treat 25% of the U.S. population should a pandemic occur in the U.S.— which is only half of the stockpile recommended in the new study in *Nature*. To date, the U.S. government has ordered 26 million antiviral treatment courses (only a fraction has been delivered), and expects to have on hand a total of 81 million treatment courses by the end of 2008.

Do the Math

It is expected that multiple courses — two or more treatments — will be required per-person, so 81 million treatment courses may treat a maximum of 40 million people, but probably fewer. The U.S. government estimates that 45 million people with H5N1 will need medical care (see Chapter 5). <u>What will the millions of people who need anti-virals — and do not get them — do?</u>

Take the matter of protecting you and your family into your own hands. Start you natural immune-optimizing regimen today (see Strategy #2 in Chapter 3), and prepare for the worst (see Chapter 5).

Novel Anti-Inflammatory Approaches

A controversial theory submits that influenza — including bird flu — causes serious illness and death in patients with an otherwise normal immune response because the immune response to the virus goes into overdrive, causing inflammation — most critically, of organs and tissues, that become overwhelmed with blood and fluids. In many cases, it is a hyper-inflammation of lung tissue that kills those who contract influenza. Additionally, cardiovascular complications from flu can result in death. Because of their potent anti-inflammatory effect, drugs approved for cardiovascular disease are now being investigated for a potential role in the prevention and/or treatment of bird flu.

ACE Inhibitors & ARBs (Angiotensin II Receptor Blockers)

The theory holds that by blocking angiotensin II, an early signal that activates the immune response (and triggers inflammation in-general), scientists may be able to modulate the immune system so it responds properly — but not overaggresively — to influenza viruses.

For more than twenty years, a variety of medications that block angiotensin II have been available. These include:

- Angiotensin I-converting enzyme (ACE) inhibitors, which prevent angiotensin I into converting into the active signal angiotensin II). Some prescription medications of this class include (brand names may vary from country to country):
  - Ramipril (Altace)
  - Quinapril (Accupril)
  - Trandolapril (Mavik)
- Angiotensin II receptor blockers (ARBs). Some prescription medications in this class include (brand names may vary from country to country):
  - Candesartan (Atacand)
  - Eprosartan (Teveten)
  - Irbesartan (Avapro)
  - Losartan (Cozaar)
  - Olmesartan (Benicar)
  - Telmisartan (Micardis)
  - Valsartan (Diovan)

There is now a clinical trial underway to evaluate the effectiveness of ACE inhibitors and ARBs to prevent the flu and/or limit the symptoms of people who get the flu. As an open trial, the study coordinators have asked interested individuals to consult their primary care physician to ask about starting an ACE inhibitor or ARB for these purposes. Certain individuals (those on immunosuppresive medications, people with diseases that cause immunosuppression, and those who have had an allergic reaction to an ARB) are excluded from the study. On a monthly basis via email, the study coordinators will conduct a survey of each study participant's overall health, and ask more specific questions if any participant contracted the flu during that month.

Expert Insight: "In avian influenza, you suffocate in pus. [ACE inhibitors and ARBs may] treat avian influenza"

David Moskowitz, MD is Chairman, CEO, and chief Medical Officer of GenoMed, Inc. (St. Louis, Missouri USA; www.genomed.com). Academically trained in internal medicine, biochemistry, and nephrology, since 1994 Dr. Moskowitz has experienced first-hand the clinical effectiveness of knowing a disease-associated gene (the angiotensin converting enzyme, or ACE, gene). The following is an excerpt from an interview conducted by Dr. Ronald Klatz with Dr. Moskowitz; you are invited to visit www.worldhealth.net/pandemic to listen to the entire interview.

Dr. Ronald Klatz: Dr. Moskowitz is world renowned as a research physician and is actively involved in exploring new applications for ACE inhibitor drugs, angiotensin blocking drugs for many purposes, some of which are preventive medicine in nature and others are infectious diseases in nature. May be you can you explain a little bit of your background and the research that your company is working on right now?

Dr. David Moskowitz: Angiotensin-I converting enzyme or ACE just converts angiotensin-I, which is a 10-amino-acid molecule and clips off the final two amino acids, so it becomes an 8-amino acid hormone called angiotensin-II. So, ACE just converts angiotensin-I into angiotensin-II.

RK: Where does this occur in the body?

DM: ACE is in a lot of places. Most importantly, it lines the vasculature. So, endothelial cells, the lining of the blood vessels, stick ACE out of their membrane. It looks like ACE is very important in keeping the circulation going. ACE is actually on white cells, on macrophages, and on immune cells. When macrophages get activated, they actually stick ACE up out their plasma membrane just like endothelial cells where it is called CD 143 and it looks like ACE is an important player in the early steps of activating immune cells.

[Within the immune system] I'm interested in are macrophages, which when they are circulating around in the blood steam are called monocytes, then they get activated [as a result of coming into contact with an allergen … a virus or something that should not be in the blood; they get ready to do battle]. They are the first line of defense against viruses and they are essentially the Generals for the innate immune response. Macrophages are even more ancient than T-cells and B-cells. They are another form of white cell.

What is important is that in viral diseases, it is actually these macrophages that fill up the organ. So, in SARS for example, in influenza — avian influenza, the lungs actually fill up with these macrophages. [W]hen your air sacs fill up with cells, you can't do gas exchange. You suffocate in pus.

(continued)

Expert Insight with Dr. David Moskowitz *(continued)*

RK: How is it that ACE inhibitor drugs and ARBs (angiotensin-II receptor blockers) might be helpful in treating avian flu?]

DM: The ACE inhibitors have been around for 30 years. The first one was captopril, and they all end in "pril." So, after captopril, there was enalapril. There is quinapril. There is trandolapril. The branded names for some of these, while quinapril is generic already but its branded name used to be Accupril, and trandolapril is a nice ACE inhibitor. It's still branded under the name of Mavik. They should work but the thing about people with viral pneumonias is that, they are probably going have low blood pressures and so we need to talk about the next class of angiotensin-II blocking agents called ARBs, angiotensin-II receptor blockers.

Angiotensin-II receptor blockers lead off with a drug called Cozaar or the generic name is losartan, and they all end in "sartan." The branded names are things like, well besides Cozaar, there is Avapro, which chemical name is irbesartan, which is actually approved for use in children. There is a drug called Atacand or candesartan, Benicar or olmesartan. There are actually seven of these drugs. They are also branded. None of them are generic yet. It's actually the ARBs, these angiotensin-II receptor blockers that we have been using for another viral illness, West Nile virus encephalitis with good effect. Clinically, if you are in coma from West Nile virus encephalitis usually, it takes four or five days to wake up from coma. We are giving people with West Nile virus coma encephalitis, we are giving them drugs like losartan or Benicar, Cozaar and they are waking up as early as 12 hours after their first dose. It doesn't take more than two days. So, within half-a-day to two days, they are already waking up, and they are completely normal. One guy woke up 12 hours after his dose of Cozaar and was working on his laptop the next morning. This is not the kind of behavior that people with viral encephalitis usually show.

RK: Have you used this with any flu or pneumonia conditions as well?

DM: We would like to, but we have not been able to. In fact, it should work for almost any virus. The only virus is that we don't think it's going to work for are the Herpes viruses. So, it is not going to work for shingles or for herpes encephalitis, or for CMV. We know it won't work for people who are immunosuppressed like transplants, people who have gotten the kidney transplant who are on high dose prednisone or cyclosporin. We know already that it won't work them but for the general population, who are immunocompetent, it should work, and for most viruses other than the herpes viruses it should work.

RK: So, what you have is, you have a drug which has been clinically available for the last 30 years that has proven its value in hypertensive patients and has actually improved longevity. May be you could explain how that works?

(continued)

Expert Insight with Dr. David Moskowitz *(continued)*

DM: We have found that besides the kidney failure [due to ACE], there were a lots of other diseases that were associated with higher activity of this enzyme, meaning that these are diseases that should get better if you use an ACE inhibitor. So, not just kidney failure from hypertension and diabetes, but all the complications of hypertension and diabetes like heart failure, strokes, coronary artery disease, peripheral vascular disease, eye disease, retinopathy and diabetes. So, that was exciting, because it meant that overactivity of ACE was behind all cardiovascular diseases. … [T]o put ACE in its proper context, we think it is one of the major aging genes. The ability to treat avian influenza just happens to be a kind of a nice corollary of ACE's widespread use in the body.

[Very few people look] at avian influenza as an overreaction of the immune system. Most people in classical virology think that the best thing you can do to the immune system is enhance it and try to jack it up, amp it up with things like interferon. [The group in Asia that] coined the phrase "cytokine storm" … is thinking the same thing, and [as well as the researcher] at the CDC who dug up people buried in the Alaskan permafrost who died of the 1918 flu virus and reconstituted that virus in the fall, just a few months ago. He also believes that virus was uniquely able to mobilize the host immune system, and essentially cause a cytokine storm.

RK: If that is the case, then shouldn't this condition be treated as acute respiratory failure with corticosteroids to modulate the inflammation and the immune system?

DM: I think you are absolutely right. That's the right track. The issue though is that acute respiratory distress syndrome, we think, it is just overactivity of ACE. There is no organ in the body that has more ACE than the lung. We think the reason is because ACE actually itself is an enzyme mediates this matching of ventilation and perfusion. When there is no oxygen that ACE gets activated, makes angiotensin to cause constriction of the blood vessels to that particular alveolus or the air sac, and shuts down blood to a nonproductive alveolus. So, given that ACE is so important in physiology, we also think that ACE is absolutely critical for pulmonary pathology too, and that it should be useful not just for avian influenza and regular influenza, pneumonia but also for other causes of acute respiratory distress syndrome like smoke inhalation.

RK: Very interesting, and this is fascinating stuff. The amazing thing is, again we have a drug that has been in common clinical use for the last 30 years with an excellent safety record. We have a drug that is readily available, that has a strong safety record, and that really, I think, deserves a much greater exploration.
Have there been any deaths associated with appropriate use of ACE inhibitors?

DM: No. No deaths that I know of, and it is being used now for 30 years by hundreds of millions of patients. I think it's much safer than aspirin.

Visit www.worldhealth.net/pandemic to listen to the entire interview with Dr. Moskowitz

Statin Drugs

The class of drugs known as statins lower levels of low-density lipoproteins — LDL ("bad") — cholesterol in people at-risk for cardiovascular complications due to hypercholesteremia (elevated cholesterol). The statins include, in alphabetical order (brand names may vary from country to country):

- Atorvastatin (Lipitor, Torvast)
- Cerivastatin (Lipobay, Baycol) [Withdrawn from the market in 2001 due to risk of serious adverse effects]
- Fluvastatin (Lescol)
- Lovastatin (Mevacor, Altocor)
- Mevastatin, a naturally-occurring compound, found in red yeast rice.
- Pitavastatin (Livalo, Pitava)
- Pravastatin (Pravachol, Selektine, Lipostat)
- Rosuvastatin (Crestor)
- Simvastatin (Zocor, Lipex)

Statins block the enzyme (HMG-CoA reductase) necessary for the body to manufacture cholesterol. This lowers intracellular cholesterol levels, and consequently causes the liver cells to increase the clearance of LDL from the bloodstream.

Statins have now been shown to reduce inflammation and help regulate the immune system. Because influenza is associated with inflammation and an increased risk of cardiovascular diseases, researchers postulate that statins confer potent anti-inflammatory and immunomodulatory effects that may be useful in preventing serious complications and death from the flu.

The most important advantage of statins for the treatment of bird flu is their ease of availability. Observes Dr. David Fedson, a retired former director of medical affairs for a major vaccine maker: "As generics, [statins] … should be available and affordable in almost all countries. For influenza, [statins] probably would be taken for only five to 10 days, and this would not have a major impact on ordinary production and sales levels by the manufacturers." Dr. Fedson notes that statins "could become the only currently available agents to alter the course of what otherwise might become an unprecedented global health crisis."

Pandemic: Not a question of *"if,"* but *"when"* ...
English Clergyman Thomas Fuller (1608-1661) remarked: "In fair weather prepare for foul." A prudent individual will prepare for disaster before it is on the doorstep.

Log on to **www.worldhealth.net/pandemic** every week to read the latest tips for protecting yourself and your loved ones from the wrath of an impending infectious disease outbreak.

Expert Insight: Statin drugs as a "potentially preventative measure [for] bird flu pandemic"

Joe Garcia, MD is the Lowell T. Coggeshall Professor and Chairman of the Department of Medicine in the University of Chicago, a leading authority on lung biology and disease, the genetics prevention and treatment of pulmonary edema and the molecular biology of blood vessels. He discusses his work in investigating the use of statin drugs for the reduction of inflammation and vascular permeability. The following is an excerpt from an interview conducted by Dr. Ronald Klatz with Dr. Garcia; you are invited to visit www.worldhealth.net/pandemic to listen to the entire interview.

Dr. Ronald Klatz: In you understanding, what is going on in the biology of these killer influenzas, whether it be annual influenza or SARS or avian influenza, what's really going on with the biology here? How does it exactly kill?

Dr. Joe Garcia: It's obviously multifactorial but a cardinal feature of the syndrome, and a cardinal feature of the morbidity and mortality is the fact that the virus induces a robust inflammatory response in the lungs, and because the immune system is not geared towards dampening that response in a timely fashion, inflammation proceeds in an unchecked manner. One the features of inflammation per se is vascular permeability or a leakiness of the blood vessels in the lung. The lungs flood with fluid as a result of this leakiness of the blood vessels and the patient's work of breathing increases to such a dramatic extent that these patients need to go on the ventilator. When the flooding is so profound and the inflammation so unchecked that even the ventilators are unable to provide this sort of oxygenation for the patient and the respiratory support and other systems start to fail and the patient expires.

RK: [If corticosteroids won't help,] [w]hat can quash the cascade of the inflammation?

JG: As far as the vascular leak, up until recently, there has been a very little hope that we might be able to come up with therapies for reducing the vascular leak that leads to flooding of the lungs. But, I think we are getting closer to some novel therapies. I will give you one example that has not been tried, and certainly in bird flu or in pandemics, but in preclinical studies, it seems to have some potential for reducing vascular leak. It is the class of drugs known as the statins. Statins have an antiinflammatory effect. The statins as everyone knows, were designed to reduce cholesterol but have been found to have profound effects on all sorts of other biological processes and by and large very beneficial effects. I think one of those biological processes might be an ability to attenuate the inflammatory response seen in viral pneumonias and other similar inflammatory syndromes.

If you are thinking about a worldwide pandemic, the availability of class of drugs like the statins should not prove to be problematic. So, whether these drugs work well after you have established inflammatory respiratory failure in older patients, nobody knows the answers to those, but certainly it is a potentially preventative measure as the bird flu

(continued)

Expert Insight with Dr. Joe Garcia *(continued)*

pandemic might ensue. It strikes me that this ought to be something that seriously considered.

My own research group is being focussed on how to control vascular permeability in the critically ill for a very long time. I do think that we are on the verge of some breakthroughs with different complementary approaches that might be able to do that. Our thinking of course is that, when you have a patient that is on a ventilator, the ventilator can also exacerbate inflammation in the lung, so that the shorter the time you are on the ventilator, the better off you are - no matter what the cause of your respiratory failure. So, we are very interested in coming up with new modalities that will stop the leakiness of the vasculature, allow the lung to resorb the fluids that are flooding the airspaces and therefore, reduce some morbidity and mortality associated with inflammatory syndromes like the bird flu.

RK: With regard to the statins, which ones have been studied, which particular forms of the statins?

JG: Simvastatin is the one that we have studied the most but other than finding differences in concentrations, the statins effects really as a class are fairly superimposable. I do not think that there is, at least in the work that we are doing, we haven't found that there is any great advantage of one of the statins over the others.

RK: Is it high-dose statins or regular dose or low dose?

JG: It's actually a reasonably low-dose. So, patient concentrations are in the sort of the 20-40 mg [per day] range. We use similar concentrations in the animal models that we are using and find very profound effects.

RK: It would be a Godsend if that were the case because there is certainly enough statins to go around. There are plenty out there.

JG: That's what our thought is. Again, I think, as you are trying to organize response teams, it would be worthwhile to conduct some studies to demonstrate that premedication with the statin, as an area becomes exposed to the bird flu may in fact have a significant effect in saving lives.

Visit www.worldhealth.net/pandemic to listen to the entire interview with Dr. Garcia

Chapter 5. Preparedness

Take Charge

Calling the arrival of H5N1 to American soil "increasingly likely," U.S. Department of the Interior Secretary Gale Norton announced a sharp increase in the testing of migratory birds to "expand our early warning system." Despite such measures, U.S. Health and Human Services Secretary Mike Leavitt urged local governments to make their own preparations for a possible human pandemic. He warned: "Any community that fails to prepare, with the expectation that the federal government will at the last moment come to the rescue, will be tragically wrong."

Michael Osterholm, the Director of Infectious Disease Research and Policy at the University of Minnesota observes that: "Most of the federal government right now is as ill-prepared as any part of society."

Consequently, it is not only important for us to heed the instructions of the federal plans for pandemic preparedness and response, but to make our own plans — for us as individuals and families — to reinforce our readiness.

Disruptions of Daily Life

In a pandemic, everyday life as we know it will suddenly halt. In its place we may find that:
- Social disruption may be widespread:
  - Usual services may be disrupted. These could include services provided by hospitals and other health care facilities, banks, stores, restaurants, government offices, and post offices.
  - Public gatherings may be canceled. These could include volunteer meetings and worship services.
  - Consider how to care for people with special needs in case the services they rely on are not available.
- Being able to work may be difficult or impossible:
  - Find out if you can work from home.
  - Ask your employer about how business will continue during a pandemic.
    - A Business Pandemic Influenza Planning Checklist is available at www.pandemicflu.gov/plan/businesschecklist.html.
  - Plan for the possible reduction or loss of income if you are unable to work or your place of employment is closed.

- Check with your employer or union about leave policies.
- Schools may be closed for an extended period of time:
  - Before a pandemic occurs, talk to the school nurse or the health center, and teachers, administrators, and parent-teacher organizations as well.
  - Plan home learning activities and exercises. Have materials, such as books, on hand. Also plan recreational activities that your children can do at home.
  - Consider childcare needs.
- Transportation services may be disrupted:
  - Presume reduced availability of public transportation. Store food and other essential supplies so you don't have to purchase these during the height of the crisis.
  - Prepare backup plans for taking care of loved ones who are far away.
  - Consider alternative ways to get to work, or, if you can, work at home.

Planning and Response at the Federal Level

The following assumptions, based largely on the 1918 influenza epidemic, are being used throughout the federal government to define a severe case scenario with regard to a potential H5N1 pandemic:

- Susceptibility to the pandemic influenza virus will be universal.
- The clinical disease attack rate will likely be 30% or higher in the overall population during the pandemic. Illness rates will be highest among school-aged children (about 40%) and decline with age. Among working adults, an average of 20% will become ill during a community outbreak.
- Risk groups for severe and fatal infection cannot be predicted with certainty but are likely to include infants, the elderly, pregnant women, and persons with chronic medical conditions.
- Persons who become ill may shed virus and can transmit infection for up to one day before the onset of illness. Viral shedding and the risk of transmission will be greatest during the first 2 days of illness. Children usually shed the greatest amount of virus and therefore are likely to post the greatest risk for transmission.
- On average, infected persons will transmit infection to approximately two other people.
- In an affected community, a pandemic outbreak will last about 6 to 8 weeks.
- Multiple waves (periods during which community outbreaks occur across the country) of illness could occur with each wave lasting 2-3 months. Historically, the largest waves have occurred in the fall and winter, but the seasonality of a pandemic cannot be predicted with certainty.

The U.S. federal government issued these projections on the medical impact of an H5N1 pandemic, in both "moderate" (similar what occurred in 1958/68) and "severe" (similar to the 1918 pandemic):

Characteristic	H5N1 – Moderate Scenario (1957/58-like)	H5N1 – Severe Scenario (1918-like)
Illness	90 million (30%)	90 million (30%)
Outpatient Medical Care	45 million (50%)	45 million (50%)
Hospitalization	865,000	9,900,000
ICU Care	128,750	1,485,000
Mechanical Ventilation	64,875	745,500
Deaths	209,000	1,903,000

NOTES:
- These estimates are based on extrapolation from past pandemics in the United States.
- These estimates do not include the potential impact of interventions (such as new antiviral medicines, see Chapter 4) not available during the 20th century pandemics.

In short, these projections demonstrate that the U.S. federal government is bracing for a "worst-case scenario" of more than 1.9 million American deaths in an H5N1 pandemic. That number is greater than the total deaths caused in a single year by heart disease, cancers, strokes, chronic pulmonary disease, AIDS, and Alzheimer's Disease combined.

The National Strategy for Pandemic Influenza

The National Strategy for Pandemic Influenza, issued by President Bush November 1, 2005, aims to guide U.S. preparedness and response to an influenza pandemic. It has three specific goals:

1. To stop, slow, or otherwise limit the spread of a pandemic to the United States
2. To limit the domestic spread of a pandemic, and mitigate disease, suffering and death
3. To sustain infrastructure and mitigate impact to the economy and the functioning of society

The World Health Network
www.worldhealth.net
The Official Website of the American Academy of Anti-Aging Medicine (A4M)
The Internet's Leading Anti-Aging Portal

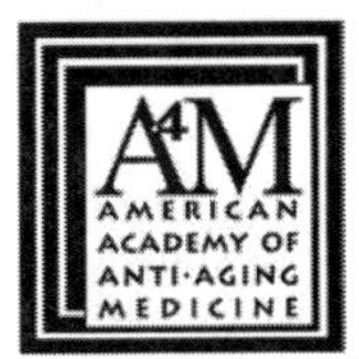

The National Strategy is comprised of three major principles, called pillars:
- Pillar One: Preparedness and Communication — Defining activities that should be undertaken before a pandemic to ensure preparedness, and the communication of roles and responsibilities to all levels of government, segments of society and individuals.
- Pillar Two: Surveillance and Detection — Establishing domestic and international systems that provide continuous "situational awareness," to ensure the earliest warning possible to protect the population.
- Pillar Three: Response and Containment — Defining actions to limit the spread of the outbreak and to mitigate the health, social and economic impacts of a pandemic.

For a copy of the 395-page National Strategy for Pandemic Influenza, visit: http://www.whitehouse.gov/homeland/pandemic-influenza.html.

Implementation Plan for the National Strategy for Pandemic Influenza

Released 3 May 2006, the Implementation Plan identifies more than 300 critical actions to effect the National Strategy. The Implementation Plan provides a common frame of reference for understanding the pandemic threat and summarizes key planning considerations for all public and private stakeholders. It also requires that Federal departments and agencies take specific coordinated steps to achieve the goals of the Strategy and outlines expectations of non-Federal stakeholders in the United States and abroad.

> The Implementation Plan assumes that 30% of the population — 100 million — would be infected, and that anywhere between 200,000 and 1.9 million would die, depending on how deadly the virus turns out to be. Yet, H5N1 has been 50%+ lethal, meaning that possibly upwards of 50 million Americans may die.

The Implementation Plan provides clear direction to Federal departments and agencies, State and local governments, communities, and the private sector on the actions that must be taken to prepare for a possible pandemic across the following six functional areas:

1. International efforts — prevent and contain outbreaks abroad
2. Transportation and borders — slow the arrival and spread of a pandemic
3. Protecting human health — limit spread and mitigate illness
4. Protecting animal health — control influenza with human pandemic potential in animals
5. Law enforcement, public safety, and security — ensure civil order during a pandemic
6. Planning by institutions — protect personnel and ensure continuity of operations

To effect these six areas, four Federal Priority Actions are identified, which are to:

1. Advance international capacity for Early Warning And Response: Most notably, to advance international cooperation with regard to reporting and sharing of scientific information.
2. Limit the arrival and spread of a pandemic: Including enhanced surveillance in humans, wild birds, and poultry; to establish border and transportation safety measures, and to arrange with international partners voluntary travel limitations and screen travelers from affected areas.
3. Provide clear guidance to all stakeholders: Communications and resource allocations to state and local agencies.
4. Accelerate the development of countermeasures: Including to develop rapid, sensitive and accurate diagnostic tests; to build stockpiles of vaccine and antiviral medications; and to advance technology and production capacity for vaccine.

The Implementation Plan stresses the importance of preparedness by individuals. It specifically states that: "Individuals Must Actively Participate. Simple infection-control measures including hand washing and staying home when ill are critical. Individuals should actively participate in their communities' responses." Reports the Plan: "It is important for U.S. citizens to recognize and understand the degree to which their actions will govern the course of a pandemic. [T]he collective response of 300 million U.S. citizens will significantly influence the shape of the pandemic and its medical, social, and economic outcomes."

For a copy of the 234 -page Implementation Plan, visit: http://www.whitehouse.gov/homeland/nspi_implementation.pdf.

HHS Plan

The National Strategy charges the U.S. Department of Health & Human Services (HHS) with leading the federal pandemic preparedness. Consequently, the HHS drafted its Pandemic Influenza Plan as a blueprint that provides guidance to national, state, and local policy makers and health departments, with the goal of achieving a state of readiness and quick response.

The HHS Plan specifies needs and opportunities to build robust preparedness for and response to pandemic influenza. Major components of the critical preparedness and ready response actions include:

- Intensifying surveillance and collaborating on containment measures – both international and domestic
- Stockpiling of antivirals and vaccines and working with industry to expand capacity for production of these medical countermeasures
- Creating a seamless network of Federal, state and local preparedness, including increasing health care surge capacity

- Developing the public education and communications efforts that will be so critical to keeping the public informed

For a copy of the HHS Pandemic Influenza Plan, visit http://www.hhs.gov/pandemicflu/plan/.

Individuals and Families

The HHS Plan urges that "an informed and responsive public is essential to minimizing the health effects of a pandemic and the resulting consequences to society." Further, the National Strategy for Pandemic Influenza states that: "The critical role of individuals and families in controlling a pandemic cannot be overstated. ... Individual action is perhaps the most important element of pandemic preparedness and response."

The National Strategy specifically makes note that: "Education on pandemic preparedness for the population should begin before a pandemic. Responsibilities of the individual and families include:

- Taking precautions to prevent the spread of infection to others if an individual or a family member has symptoms of influenza.
- Being prepared to follow public health guidance that may include limitation of attendance at public gatherings and non-essential travel for several days or weeks.
- Keeping supplies of materials at home, as recommended by authorities, to support essential needs of the household for several days if necessary."

A severe pandemic could change the patterns of daily life for some time. People may choose to stay home to keep away from others who are sick. Also, people may need to stay home to care for ill family and loved ones. Travel and public gatherings could be limited. Basic services and access to supplies could be disrupted. At the federal government's warning, then, it is of paramount importance that each of us prepares ourselves and our families.

With the federal government presuming that:

- In an affected community, <u>a pandemic outbreak will last about 6 to 8 weeks</u>; and that
- Multiple waves (periods during which community outbreaks occur across the country) of illness could occur with <u>each wave lasting 2-3 months.</u> The 1918 pandemic consisted of 3 major waves.

<u>It is critical that each of us makes preparations — including stockpiles of supplies — to last a minimum of 6 weeks to 18 months, maybe more.</u>

Pandemic Flu Planning Checklist for Individuals and Families

1. Store items for an extended stay at-home: a two-week minimum's supply of water, food/ nonperishables, and medical, health, and emergency supplies:

- Bottled water: 2-4 gallons per person per day
- Ready-to-eat canned meats, fruits, vegetables, and soups
- Protein or fruit bars
- Dry cereal or granola
- Peanut butter or nuts
- Dried fruit
- Crackers
- Canned juices
- Canned or jarred baby food and formula
- Pet food
- Prescribed medical supplies such as glucose and blood-pressure monitoring equipment
- Nonprescription drugs and other health supplies on hand, including pain relievers (especially for fever, such as aspirin, acetaminophen and/or ibuprofen), stomach remedies (especially anti-diarrheal medication), cough and cold medicines, fluids with electrolytes, and vitamins
- Soap and water, and alcohol-based hand sanitizers
- Thermometer
- Cleansing agent/soap
- Flashlight
- Batteries
- Portable radio
- Manual can opener
- Garbage bags
- Tissues, toilet paper, disposable diapers

2. Talk with family members and loved ones about how they would be cared for if they got sick, or what will be needed to care for them in your home.
3. Volunteer with local groups to prepare and assist with emergency response.
4. Get involved in your community as it works to prepare for an influenza pandemic.

For more information on the Pandemic Flu Planning Checklist for Individuals and Families, visit: http://www.pandemicflu.gov/planguide/checklist.html.

Self Isolation

A study published in the scientific journal *Nature* in April 2006 reports on various modeling simulations to mitigate a bird flu pandemic. Of all the methods tested, the study recommends rapid treatment and quarantine of not only infected people, but also their uninfected household contacts. <u>The study found that isolation of entire households, in addition to rapid treatment with antiviral drugs, could reduce infection rates by nearly 50%.</u> The study, which was completed by the U.S. National Institute of General Medical Sciences, recommends a policy of social distancing, including the closing of schools and telling people to stay home from work.

Stock these supplies for your self isolation in the event of pandemic:
- Plastic sheeting
- Duct tape
- Self defense armaments, such as handgun or shotgun
- Citizen's band (CB) or ham radio
- Extra cellphone batteries
- Cash

Family Emergency Health Information Sheet

In the event of a pandemic, public health officials may need you to provide information about your and your family's medical history. Prepare a chart that lists the following data:
- Family Member Name
- Blood Type
- Allergies
- Past/ Current Medical Conditions
- Current Medications/ Dosages

A downloadable Family Emergency Health Information Sheet is available from: http://www.pandemicflu.gov/planguide/familyhealthinfo.html.

Emergency Contacts Form
Prepare a chart that lists telephone numbers, email addresses, and fax numbers for each of the following contacts:
- Local personal emergency contact
- Out-of-town personal emergency contact
- Hospitals near: Work; School; Home
- Family physician(s)
- State public health department (listed at www.cdc.gov/other.htm#states)
- Pharmacy
- Employer contact and emergency information
- School contact and emergency information
- Religious/spiritual organization

A downloadable Emergency Contacts Form is available from:
http://www.pandemicflu.gov/planguide/emergencycontacts.html.

The powerful positive impact of networks of friends and colleagues to share the burdens during a pandemic cannot be understated. In advance of a crisis:
- Think about what information the people in your workplace will need if you are a manager. This may include information about insurance, leave policies, working from home, possible loss of income, and when not to come to work if sick.
- Meet with your colleagues and make lists of things that you will need to know and what actions can be taken.
- Find volunteers who want to help people in need, such as elderly neighbors, single parents of small children, or people without the resources to get the medical help they will need.
- Identify other information resources in your community, such as mental health hotlines, public health hotlines, or electronic bulletin boards.
- Find support systems — people who are thinking about the same issues you are thinking about. Share ideas.

Finally, perhaps the most critical preparedness step is to get — and stay — informed. Reliable, accurate, and timely information is available from:
- The U.S. Department of Health & Human Services at www.pandemicflu.gov.
- The U.S. Centers for Disease Control and Prevention (CDC) at www.cdc.gov. They also have a phone hotline at: 800-CDC-INFO (1-800-232-4636). This line is available in English and Spanish, 24/7.
- Local and state government Web sites. Links are available to each state department of public health at www.pandemicflu.gov/plan/tab2.html.
- Local and national radio, watch news reports on television, visit Internet news sites, and read your newspaper.
- Talk to your local health care providers and public health officials.

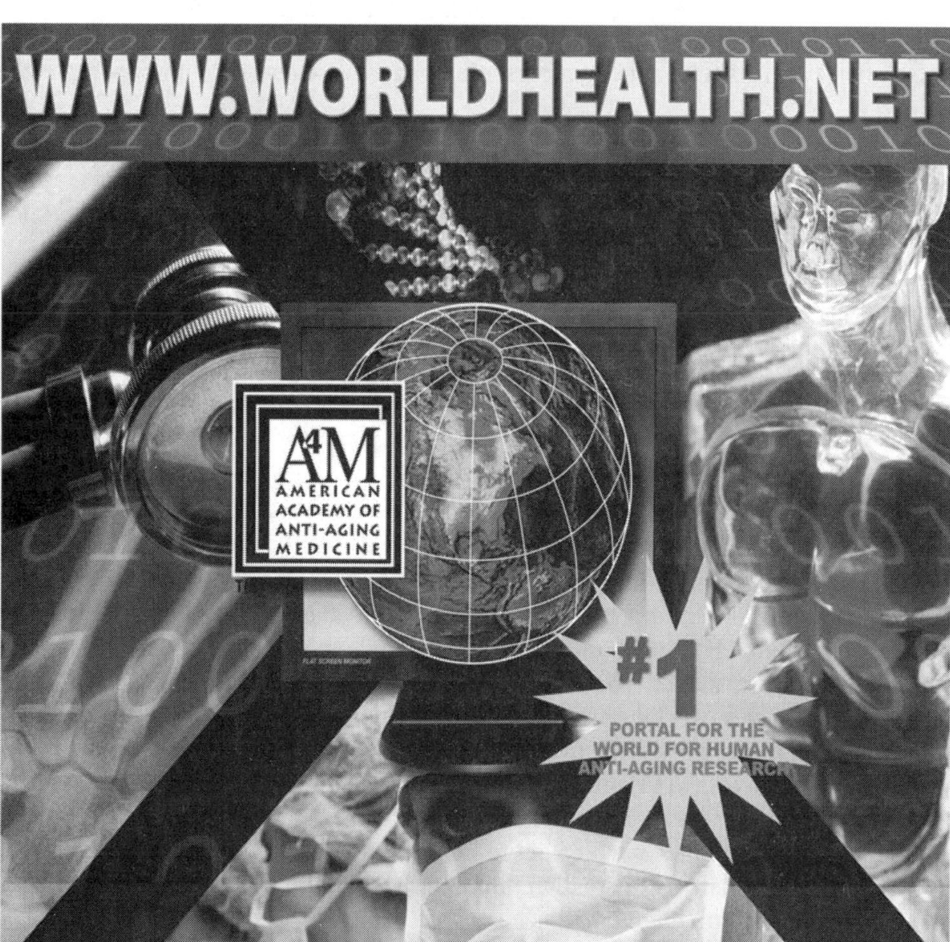
WWW.WORLDHEALTH.NET
A4M
AMERICAN ACADEMY OF ANTI-AGING MEDICINE
#1
PORTAL FOR THE WORLD FOR HUMAN ANTI-AGING RESEARCH
• Listed #1 For Anti-aging Related Keywords On Google, Yahoo, MSN, AOL And Other Major Search Engines.
• 20 Million Hits Per Month
• FREE Electronic Bio-Newsletter ($149 Value)
• World's Leading Resource Of Anti-Aging Related News
• Online Video Directory Of Physicians, Products And Services
• Archival Library Of Over 100,000 Referenced Research Papers
WWW.WORLDHEALTH.NET

Chapter 6. Vigilance

The Need for Ongoing Vigilance & Preparedness

Thanks to the advent of antibiotics, antivirals, and antimicrobial agents, many people — including public health experts — considered the longstanding battle of humans versus infectious disease as over, with humankind prevailing as the winner. However, as the U.S. National Institute of Allergy & Infectious Diseases wrote: "The events of the past two decades have shown the foolhardiness of this position."

At least a dozen "new" diseases have been identified — such as AIDS, Legionnaire's disease, hantavirus pulmonary syndrome, and severe acute respiratory syndrome (SARS). In addition, traditional diseases — such as malaria and tuberculosis — that had appeared to be trailing off, are now on the upsurge.

Globally, infectious diseases remain the leading cause of death, and they are the third leading cause of death in the United States.

The emergence and reemergence of a wide variety of disease-causing pathogens has been fueled by several factors, including:
- Unprecedented worldwide population growth
- Increased international travel
- Increasing worldwide transport of animals and food products
- Changes in food processing and handling
- Changes in human behavior
- Human encroachment on wilderness habitats that are reservoirs for insects and animals that harbor infectious agents
- Microbial evolution and the development of resistance to antibiotics and other antimicrobial drugs

Emerging Infectious Diseases

"Emerging infectious diseases" are diseases with the following characteristics:
1. they have not occurred in humans before (this type of emergence is difficult to establish);
2. they have occurred previously, but affected only small numbers of people in isolated places (examples include AIDS and Ebola hemorrhagic fever); or
3. they have occurred throughout human history but have only recently been recognized as distinct diseases due to an infectious agent (examples include Lyme disease and gastric ulcers)

Examples of emerging infectious diseases are presented on the following table:

Disease	Infectious Agent	Year Recognized (year in which infectious agent was identified)	Contributing Factors
Lassa fever	Arenavirendae family (virus)	1969	Urbanization and other conditions that favor the rodent host; transmission via hospitals or medical treatment
Ebola hemorrhagic fever	Filoviridae family (virus)	1977	Unknown natural host; transmission via hospitals or medical treatment
Legionnaire disease	Legionella pneumophila (bacterium)	1977	Cooling and plumbing system
Hemolytic uremic syndrome	Escherichia coli 0157:H7 (bacterium)	1982	Mass food production systems
Lyme borreliosis	Borrelia burgdorferi (bacterium)	1982	Conditions favoring the tick insect (mode of transmission) and deer (host)
AIDS	Human immunodeficiency virus	1983	Migration to cities, global travel, transfusions, organ transplants, intravenous drug use, multiple sexual partners
Gastric ulcers	Helicobacter pylori (bacterium)	1983	
			(continued)

Cholera	Vibrio cholerae 0139 (bacterium)	1992	Evolution of new strain of bacteria combining increased virulence and long-term survival in environment
Hantavirus pulmonary syndrome	Bunyaviridae family (virus)	1993	Environmental changes favoring contact with rodent hosts
Pandemic influenza	Orthomyxoviridae family (virus)	New viral strains emerge periodically	Pig-duck agriculture (possible mechanism)
Source: Understanding Emerging and Re-Emerging Infectious Diseases, U.S. National Institute of Allergy and Infectious Diseases, October 1999. From Morse, S.S. 1995. Factors in the emergence of infectious diseases. *Emerging Infectious Diseases* [Serial online], 1(1). Available http://www.cdc.gov/ncidod/EID/index.htm. June 1999; Satcher, D. 1995. Emerging infections: Getting ahead of the curve. *Emerging Infectious Diseases* [Serial online], 1(1). Available http://www.cdc.gov/ncidod/EID/index.htm. June 1999; Morse, S.S. (Ed.). 1993. Examining the origins of emerging viruses. *Emerging viruses.* New York: Oxford University Press; ProMED. 1994. About ProMED. Available http:// www.fas.org/promed/about/index.html, June 1999.			

The above table suggests two primary themes in the emergence of new infectious diseases:

1. Environmental changes contribute to the emergence of many infectious diseases. Lyme disease, emerged when humans began encountering the insect responsible for transmission; both hantavirus pulmonary syndrome and Lassa fever emerged as a result of increased contact with the host rodent animal.
2. The large-scale introduction of modern technologies caused Legionnaire to emerge (air conditioning) as well as hemolytic uremic syndrome (mass food production systems).

Pandemic: Not a question of *"if,"* but *"when"* ...
English Clergyman Thomas Fuller (1608-1661) remarked: "In fair weather prepare for foul." A prudent individual will prepare for disaster before it is on the doorstep.

Log on to **www.worldhealth.net/pandemic** every week to read the latest tips for protecting yourself and your loved ones from the wrath of an impending infectious disease outbreak.

SARS

Severe acute respiratory syndrome (SARS) is a viral respiratory illness caused by a coronavirus, called SARS-associated coronavirus (SARS-CoV). The main way that SARS seems to spread is by close person-to-person contact. The virus that causes SARS is thought to be transmitted most readily by respiratory droplets (droplet spread) produced when an infected person coughs or sneezes. Droplet spread can happen when droplets from the cough or sneeze of an infected person are propelled a short distance (generally up to 3 feet [1 meter]) through the air and deposited on the mucous membranes of the mouth, nose, or eyes of persons who are nearby. The virus also can spread when a person touches a surface or object contaminated with infectious droplets and then touches his or her mouth, nose, or eye(s). The World Health Organization (WHO) also has suggested that inadequate plumbing and sewage systems are likely to have contributed to the spread of SARS. Droplets originating from virus-rich fecal excrements in a building's drainage system could re-enter another apartment in the same building via sewage and drainage systems where there were strong upward air flows, inadequate "traps" and non-functional water seals.

SARS was first reported in Asia in February 2003. According to the World Health Organization (WHO), a total of 8,098 people worldwide became sick with SARS during the 2003 outbreak. Of these, 774 died. During the course of the epidemic, SARS spread to more than two dozen countries in North America, South America, Europe, and Asia before the SARS global outbreak of 2003 was contained.

In the United States, only eight people had laboratory evidence of SARS-CoV infection. All of these people had traveled to other parts of the world with SARS. Fortunately, SARS did not spread more widely in the community in the United States.

At present, there is no vaccine for SARS, and the WHO noted in the fall of 2003 that: "If there is no big outbreak of SARS then the vaccine will follow the classical development path, and would not be ready for four to five years."

Watching the Very Newest Threat

A little-known mosquito-borne virus is spreading pain and death across the Indian Ocean, and could be headed for Europe and the Americas. So far, the Chikungunya virus has not been fatal and large outbreaks have been rare. Now, however, the virus has crossed the Indian Ocean and struck one-third of the population of the French island of Reunion in the first quarter of 2006 with deadly consequences.

The mosquitoes that carry the Chikungunya virus are now invading Europe and the Americas, and there are early signs that the virus could have already reached these previously unaffected regions.

The chief characteristic symptom of Chikungunya is excruciating pain in the small joints of the body, which gives the disease the nickname "knuckle fever." The virus also causes fever, headache, nausea and a rash. The pain usually lasts just a few days, but in some cases the pain and stiffness can persist for months — even years.

Re-Emerging infectious Diseases

"Re-emerging infectious diseases" are diseases that once were major health problems globally or in a particular country, then declined dramatically, but are again becoming health problems for a large segment of the population.

Examples of re-emerging infectious diseases are presented on the following table:

Disease	Infectious Agent	Contributing Factors
Cryptosporidiosis	Cryptosporidium parvum (protozoa)	Inadequate control in water supply; international travel; increased use of child-care facilities
Diphtheria	Corynebacterium diptheriae (bacteria)	Interruption of immunization program due to political changes
Malaria	Plasmodium species (protozoon)	Drug resistance; favorable conditions for mosquito (mode of transmission)
Meningitis, necrotizing fasciitis (flesh-eating disease), toxic shock syndrome, and other diseases	Group A Streptococcus (bacterium)	
Pertussis (whooping cough)	Bordetella pertussis (bacterium)	Refusal to vaccinate based on fears about vaccine safety; decreased vaccine efficacy; waning immunity among vaccinated adults
Rabies	Rhabdovirus group (virus)	Breakdown in public health measures; changes in land use; travel
Rubeola (measles)	Morbillivirus genus (virus)	Failure to vaccinate; failure to receive second dose of vaccine
Schistosomiasis	Schistosoma species (helminth)	Dam construction; ecological changes favoring snail host
		(continued)

Tuberculosis	Mycobacterium tuberculosis (bacterium)	Antibiotic-resistant pathogens; immunocompromised populations (malnourished, HIV-infected, poverty-stricken)
Yellow fever	Flavivirus group (virus)	Insecticide resistance; urbanization; civil strife

Source: Understanding Emerging and Re-Emerging Infectious Diseases, U.S. National Institute of Allergy and Infectious Diseases, October 1999. From Krause, R.M. 1992. The origin of plagues: Old and new. *Science, 257*: 1073-1078; Measles—United States, 1997. April 17, 1998. *Morbidity and Mortality Weekly Report, 47*(14): 273-276; Pertussis vaccination: Use of acellular pertussis vaccines among infants and young children. 1997, March 28. *Morbidity and Mortality Weekly Report, 46*(RR-7); ProMED. 1994. About ProMED. Available from http://www.fas.org/promed/about/index.html. June 1999.

As the above table suggests, prominent themes in the re-emergence of infectious diseases include:

1. Evolution of the causative pathogen: Both tuberculosis and malaria have re-emerged due to a newfound drug resistance by the organisms that cause these diseases.
2. Inadequate vaccination of the population: Contributing to the rise in diphtheria and whooping cough. If the proportion of immune individuals in a population drops below a threshold, an outbreak of the disease may occur.

In early 2006, a mumps outbreak occurred in the United States. Mumps, an infection caused by the mumps virus, s spread by mucus or droplets from the nose or throat of an infected person, usually when a person coughs or sneezes. Surfaces of items can also spread the virus if someone who is sick touches them without washing their hands, and someone else then touches the same surface and then rubs their eyes, mouth, or nose. The first cases of mumps-like illness in the recent outbreak were reported from Iowa in December 2005. Airline travel of two people diagnosed with mumps in the state of Iowa may have resulted with the infection spreading to affect people in Arkansas, Colorado, Iowa, Illinois, Kansas, Mississippi, Missouri, Minnesota, Nebraska, New York, Pennsylvania, South Dakota, and Wisconsin.

In mid-2006, a measles outbreak occurred in Massachusetts, where 11 cases have been reported as of this writing. Measles is the <u>most infectious</u> human disease. Infectious particles can remain suspended in the air for up to 2 hours. Measles is transmitted from person-to-person by droplet, direct contact and the airborne route. The infectious period is from 4 days before to 4 days after rash onset (counting the rash onset as day zero). In Massachusetts, the index case in the recent outbreak occurred in a 32 year old unvaccinated man who arrived from India in April 2006, and 7 of the other 11 cases to-date are of individuals who work in the same building as the initial case. In the United Kingdom, the number of measles cases has reached a record-breaking high in 20 years. Compared to 2005 when England and Wales had 77 cases of measles, by midyear 2006 the English counties of Surrey and Sussex reported 156 cases with South Yorkshire reporting 180.

The ability of diseases previously thought to have been eliminated to so robustly re-emerge provides clear reason that each of us should not be complacent in the ongoing battle against infectious pathogens. The reemergence of pathogenic disease on a pandemic scale is frighteningly real, and, as authors of this book, we hope you have learned some important ways to optimize your immune system in-preparation for what lies ahead.

Concluding Thoughts on Bird Flu

Infection Protection: Pandemic was written by leading anti-aging medical physicians in order to help you succeed in upholding the Three Rules of Anti-Aging Medicine, namely:

Rule #1. Don't Get Sick
Rule #2. Don't Get Old
Rule #3. Don't Die

A key way to avoid violating Rules #1 and #3 is by not succumbing to infectious diseases. To achieve Rule #2, seek guidance from a qualified anti-aging physician who can design a well-rounded preventive health regimen specifically for your health needs.

As authors of *Infection Protection: Pandemic* and leaders in the anti-aging movement, we submit that there exist dozens — perhaps hundreds — of unknown and unexploited methods of halting H5N1 and many other viral diseases, which require consolidation and cataloguing to put them to use:

1. Federally funded research into bioresponse technologies have yielded dozens of secret or otherwise unreported preventive and interventive protocols, which — for the good of the nation's health — must be released and made public.

2. Dozens — if not hundreds — of non-toxic antiviral substances known in non-mainstream medicine (such as Ayurvedic and Traditional Chinese medicine systems) have hundreds to thousands of years of proven efficacy.

3. The fields of naturopathic, nutritional, and herbal medicine offer hundreds of natural compounds with proven track records in warding off Spanish Flu, SARS, etc., and have the same potential for H5N1. Regrettably, knowledge of these interventions is marginalized due to the dominating premise in infectious disease research that proprietary agents or vaccines that are owned at-profit by multinational pharmaceutical corporations are superior to natural remedies. Many of the entries listed in this book's "Immunity Desk Reference" (see Chapter 3) offer real potential for counteracting H5N1, but require more comprehensive study at an expedited pace.

4. Methods of protecting personal space, hands, and face, including antiviral aseptic gloves and other protective gear, are simple, effective, and

inexpensive ways to avoid contagion contact that should also be further elucidated.

Any one of the protocols or technologies listed above may be responsible for saving hundreds of millions of dollars and tens of thousands of lives.   More interestingly, the bird flu virus has yet to be specifically identified, isolated, cultured, and proven to be virulent to humankind. As the authors of *Infection Protection: Pandemic,* we hope that this book will stimulate action to expedite research and implementation of innovative, safe, and effective preventive and interventive methods for bird flu.

What YOU Need to Do

With regard to preparedness for natural disasters, in June 2006, the U.S. Department of Homeland Security issued a report that found major shortcomings in many cities and states in the arena of emergency planning that are cause for significant national concern. Despite spending $18 billion in grants to prompt local preparedness since 9|11, many local and state governments are using antiquated and uncoordinated response guidelines. Most eye-opening of all is that the Homeland Security report warns that cities including New York and Washington, DC are woefully prepared for catastrophes. Such is the case for dealing with known disasters in which we have a knowledge base of experiences (both positive and negative). What will happen if, or when, avian flu — which will present a wide array of unprecedented challenges — grips the nation?

Protect yourself and your family by preparing well in advance of any threat to your health or longevity:

1. Have an Emergency Plan, which should include:
    - Researched information as to the preparedness of your local community, county, and state in the event of any disaster — weather, medical, or otherwise
    - Inform all members of your family with this information. Collect their questions and incorporate the answers into your Emergency Plan.
    - Stock emergency supplies: a two-week minimum's supply of water, food/nonperishables, and medical, health, and emergency supplies (see Chapter 5).
    - Complete family information sheets and forms as appropriate (see Chapter 5).
    - Prepare for self-isolation if you choose to do so (see Chapter 5)
2. Practice the Top Ten strategies of:
    Strategy #1. Hygiene habits
    Strategy #2. Natural immune enhancement
    Strategy #3. Hydration
    Strategy #4. Daily nutrition
    Strategy #5. Poultry safety
    Strategy #6. Face masks and respirators

Strategy #7. Barriers
Strategy #8. Ventilation
Strategy #9. Humidification
Strategy #10. Safe and smart travel

3. Stay vigilant, at all times, to any potential threats that could compromise your health.
4. Gather information from reliable, independent sources. Reliable, accurate, and timely information is available from:

- The U.S. Department of Health & Human Services at www.pandemicflu.gov.
- The U.S. Centers for Disease Control and Prevention (CDC) at www.cdc.gov. They also have a phone hotline at: 800-CDC-INFO (1-800-232-4636). This line is available in English and Spanish, 24 hours a day, 7 days a week. TTY: 1-888-232-6348.
- Local and state government Web sites. Links are available to each state department of public health at www.pandemicflu.gov/plan/tab2.html.
- Local and national radio, watch news reports on television, visit Internet news sites, and read your newspaper.
- Talk to your local health care providers and public health officials.

Relevant Websites for Information on Bird Flu

Infection Protection: Pandemic Avian Flu Update: www.worldhealth.net/pandemic

The World Health Network, the official website of the A4M and the Internet's leading anti-aging portal: www.worldhealth.net

MyLongLife.com, an informational website on the subject of human longevity: www.mylonglife.com

U.S. Department of Health & Human Services Avian Influenza website: www.pandemicflu.gov

U.S. Centers for Disease Control & Prevention Avian Influenza webarea: http://www.cdc.gov/flu/avian/index.htm

World Health Organization Avian Influenza webarea: http://www.who.int/csr/disease/avian_influenza/en/index.html

---

Your Source for the Best Physician-Selected Products from the New Science of Anti-Aging Medicine

Physicians' picks of the "best of the best" of essential anti-aging health products — including those for immune optimization. 100% satisfaction guaranteed. Read more information about natural immune-optimizing approaches at **www.lexmd.com**.

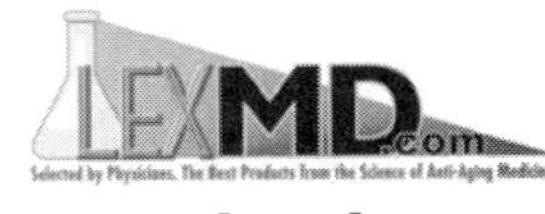

www.lexmd.com

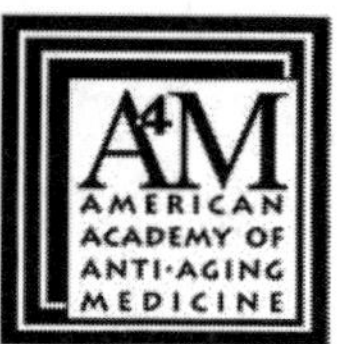

The American Academy of Anti-Aging Medicine (A4M) is the leading worldwide medical organization dedicated to the advancement of technology to detect, prevent, and treat aging related disease and to promote research into methods to retard and optimize the human aging process. As a federally registered (USA) non-profit medical organization, A4M is also dedicated to educating physicians, scientists, and members of the public on anti-aging issues. With 18,500 physician and sciensist members from 85 nations worldwide, A4M believes that the disabilities associated with normal aging are caused by physiological dysfunction which in many cases are ameliorable to medical treatment, such that the human lifespan can be increased, and the quality of one's life improved as one grows chronologically older. Through its Internet presence (**www.worldhealth.net**), publications, and scientific education programs, A4M shares information concerning innovative science and research relating to extension of the healthy human lifespan.

The Last Word

Be mindful of the following:

- Worldwide, 5 to 150 million people may die from bird flu
- Pandemic conditions will wreak havoc on everyday life, disrupting society and the economy at-large
- The U.S. government has earmarked US $7 Billion for federal preparations
- The nations of the world are stockpiling Tamiflu

It is up to you to prepare yourself — and your loved ones — for a potential H5N1 pandemic. Even if the pandemic never manifests, you'll have taken important steps to improving your overall immunity which may contribute to extending your healthy, robust, productive, fulfilling life.

Appendix A. Additional Reading, Relevant Websites, and Product Resources

ADDITIONAL READING

Klatz R. and Goldman R. *Infection Protection: How to Fight the Germs That Make You Sick.* New York: HarperCollins, 2002. Available from the American Academy of Anti-Aging Medicine (A4M); call (773) 528-4333 or visit www.worldhealth.net.

Klatz R. and Goldman R. *The New Anti-Aging Revolution.* North Bergen, NJ: Basic Health Publications, 2003. Available from the American Academy of Anti-Aging Medicine (A4M); call (773) 528-4333 or visit www.worldhealth.net.

RELEVANT WEBSITES

Infection Protection: Pandemic Avian Flu Update: www.worldhealth.net/pandemic

The World Health Network, the official website of the A4M and the Internet's leading anti-aging portal: www.worldhealth.net

MyLongLife.com, an informational website on the subject of human longevity: www.mylonglife.com

U.S. Department of Health & Human Services Avian Influenza website: www.pandemicflu.gov

U.S. Centers for Disease Control & Prevention Avian Influenza webarea: http://www.cdc.gov/flu/avian/index.htm

World Health Organization Avian Influenza webarea: http://www.who.int/csr/disease/avian_influenza/en/index.html

PRODUCT RESOURCES

As noted in the "Immunity Desk Reference" appearing in Chapter 3, we consider the Top Ten Natural Immune Enhancers to be:

- Arabinogalactan
- EpiCor™*
- Green tea
- Glutathione
- ImmunoMax*
- Inositol hexaphosphate (IP6)
- Lactoferrin
- Mushrooms (maitake, shitake)
- Oregano oil
- Selenium

*Epicor™ and ImmunoMax are available from a company called Vitamin Research Products (Carson City, NV USA; www.vrp.com). All other above-listed immune enhancers are also available from Vitamin Research Products and other dietary supplement companies.

Neem is available from www.neemwell.com.

Specialty nutritional products, including custom-compounded pharmaceuticals, are available from:

- Abrams Royal Pharmacy (Dallas, TX USA): www.abramsroyalpharmacy.com
- Applied Pharmacy Services (Mobile, AL USA): www.appliedpharmacyrx.com
- Central Drugs Compounding Pharmacy (La Habra, CA USA): www.anypharmacy.com
- College Pharmacy (Colorado Springs, CO USA): www.collegepharmacy.com
- Essential Pharmacy Compounding (Omaha, NE USA): www.kohlls.com
- Medaus Pharmacy (Birmingham, AL USA): www.medaus.com
- MedQuest Pharmacy (North Salt Lake, UT USA): www.mqrx.com
- North Shore Compounding Pharmacy (Deerfield, IL USA)
- Signature Compounding Pharmacy (Orlando, FL USA): www.signaturepharmacy.com
- University Compounding Pharmacy (San Diego, CA USA): www.ucprx.com
- Women's International Pharmacy (Madison, WI USA): www.womensinternational.com

Appendix B. Bibliography

PREFACE

Anderson RN and Smith BL. Deaths: Leading Causes for 2002. National Vital Statistics Reports, Volume 53, Number 17. http://www.cdc.gov/nchs/data/nvsr/nvsr53/nvsr53_17.pdf. Accessed 12 June 2006.

Avian flu: human pandemic, The World Bank. http://web.worldbank.org/WBSITE/EXTERNAL/EXTDEC/EXTDECPROSPECTS/EXTGBLPRO SPECTSAPRIL/0,,contentMDK:20894257~menuPK:2466750~pagePK:2470434~piPK:2470429~t heSitePK:659149,00.html. Accessed 12 June 2006.

Journal Antimicrobial Chemotherapy 55: S-1, 2005.

Kolata G. *Flu: The Story of the Great Influenza Pandemic of 1918 and the Search for the Virus that Caused It.* New York: Farrar, Straus and Giroux, 1999.

"Ten things you need to know about pandemic influenza," World Health Organization, 14 October 2005. http://www.who.int/csr/disease/influenza/pandemic10things/en/. Accessed 12 June 2006.

U.S. Centers for Disease Control & Prevention (CDC) Avian Flu website, http://www.cdc.gov/flu/avian/.

U.S. Department of Health and Human Services (HHS) Pandemic Flu website, www.pandemicflu.gov.

CHAPTER 1

"Avian flu: human pandemic," The World Bank. http://web.worldbank.org/WBSITE/EXTERNAL/EXTDEC/EXTDECPROSPECTS/EXTGBLPRO SPECTSAPRIL/0,,contentMDK:20894257~menuPK:2466750~pagePK:2470434~piPK:2470429~t heSitePK:659149,00.html. Accessed 12 June 2006.

"Cumulative Number of Confirmed Human Cases of Avian Influenza (H5N1) Reported to WHO," World Health Organization Epidemic and Pandemic Alert and Response, 6 June 2006. http://www.who.int/csr/disease/avian_influenza/country/cases_table_2006_06_06/en/index.html. Accessed 12 June 2006.

"Indonesia Situation Update," U.S. Department of Health & Human Services, May 31, 2006. http://www.pandemicflu.gov/news/indonesiaupdate.html. Accessed 12 June 2006.

"Indonesia struggles to track H5N1 source, two more die," Reuters, 22 May 2006.

J Gen Virol. 2003 Sep;84(Pt 9):2285-92. Vaccine. 2002 Aug 19;20(25-26):3068-87.

Sardi B. "What you should know about Tamiflu," 8 October 2005. http://www.knowledgeofhealth.com/report.asp?story=What%20You%20Should%20Know%20Abo ut%20Tamiflu&catagory=Infectious%20Disease,%20Vaccines,%20Flu,%20Drugs. Accessed 18 May 2006.

Siegel M. *Bird Flu: Everything You Need to Know About the Next Pandemic.* Hoboken, NJ: John Wiley & Sons, Inc., 2006.

"Ten things you need to know about pandemic influenza," World Health Organization, 14 October 2005. http://www.who.int/csr/disease/influenza/pandemic10things/en/. Accessed 12 June 2006.

U.S. Centers for Disease Control & Prevention (CDC) Avian Flu website, http://www.cdc.gov/flu/avian/.

U.S. Department of Health and Human Services (HHS) Pandemic Flu website, www.pandemicflu.gov.

CHAPTER 2

Balch P. *Prescription for Nutritional Healing, Third Edition,* 2000.

Bell JR. "Avian flu avoids upper airway, thwarting spread in humans," Internal Medicine News, 1 May 2006.

"Bird flu may infect people through the gut, virologist says," Bloomberg.com, May 9, 2006.

Fox M. "Flu vaccine recommended for more Americans in 2006-7 season," Reuters Health Information, 19 May 2006.

Griffith HW. *Complete Guide to Symptoms, Illness & Surgery, 3rd edition.* New York: The Body Press/Perigee Books, 1995.

"Has Asia eliminated bird flu," Foodconsumer.org, 14 May 2006. http://www.foodconsumer.org/777/8/Has_Asia_eliminated_bird_flu_.shtml. Accessed 16 May 2006.

"Influenza Virus A," Wikipedia.com. http://en.wikipedia.org/wiki/Influenzavirus_A. Accessed 10 June 2006.

"Outbreak: Could it happen here?," DatelineNBC, airdate 23 April 2006.

"Pandemic Planning Update," U.S. Department of Health & Human Services, 13 March 2006. http://www.pandemicflu.gov/plan/pdf/panflu20060313.pdf. Accessed 9 May 2006.

"Seasonal Flu," U.S. Centers for Disease Control & Prevention. http://www.cdc.gov/flu/. Accessed 13 June 2006.

U.S. Centers for Disease Control & Prevention (CDC) Avian Flu website, http://www.cdc.gov/flu/avian/.

U.S. Department of Health and Human Services (HHS) Pandemic Flu website, www.pandemicflu.gov.

CHAPTER 3

"Anti-Aging Desk Reference 2005," appearing in *Anti-Aging Therapeutics volume 7,* American Academy of Anti-Aging Medicine, 2005.

Araki S, Suzuki M, Fujimoto M, Kimura M. Enhancement of resistance to bacterial infection in mice by vitamin B2. J Vet Med Sci. 1995;57:599-602.

De Flora S, Grassi C, Carati L. Attenuation of influenza-like symptomatology and improvement of cell-mediated immunity with long-term N-acetylcysteine treatment. Eur Respir J. 1997;10:1535-1541.

Djeraba A, Quere P. In vivo macrophage activation in chickens with Acemannan, a complex carbohydrate extracted from Aloe vera. Int J Immunopharmacol. 2000;22:365-372.

Dorman HJ, Deans SG. Antimicrobial agents from plants: antibacterial activity of plant volatile oils. J Applied Microbiology. 2000;88:308-316.

Edelson R, Berger C, Gasparro F, Jegasothy B, Heald P, Wintroub B, Vonderheid E, Knobler R, Wolff K, Plewig G, et al. Treatment of cutaneous T-cell lymphoma by extracorporeal photochemotherapy. Preliminary results. N Engl J Med. 1987;316:297-303.

Engwerda CR, Andrew D, Murphy M, Mynott TL. Bromelain activates murine macrophages and natural killer cells in vitro. Cell Immunol. 2001;210:5-10.

Faresjo MK, Ernerudh J, Berlin G, Garcia J, Ludvigsson J. The immunological effect of photopheresis in children with newly diagnosed type 1 diabetes. Pediatr Res. 2005;58:459-466.

"FDA acts to protect public from fraudulent avian flu therapies," U.S. Food & Drug Administration, 13 December 2005.

"Fear the phone, not the doorknob, US germ expert says," Reuters, 2 May 2006.

Field CJ, Van Aerde A, Drager KL, Goruk S, Basu T. Dietary folate improves age-related decreases in lymphocyte function. J Nutr Biochem. 2006;17:37-44. Epub 2005 May 31.

Fort P, Moses N, Fasano M, Goldberg T, Lifshitz F. Breast and soy-formula feedings in early infancy and the prevalence of autoimmune thyroid disease in children. J Am Coll Nutr. 1990;9:164-167.

Galland L. Magnesium and immune function: an overview. Magnesium. 1988;7:290-299.

Gallin EK, Green SW, Patchen ML. Comparative effects of particulate and soluble glucan on macrophages of C3H/HeN and C3H/HeJ mice. Int J Immunopharmacol. 1992;14:173-183.

Glatthaar-Saalmuller B, Sacher F, Esperester A. Antiviral activity of an extract derived from roots of Eleutherococcus senticosus. Antiviral Res. 2001;50:223-228.

Goel V, Chang C, Slama JV, Barton R, Bauer R, Gahler R, Basu TK. Alkylamides of Echinacea purpurea stimulate alveolar macrophage function in normal rats. Int Immunopharmacol. 2002;2:381-387.

Gorton HC, Jarvis K. The effectiveness of vitamin C in preventing and relieving the symptoms of virus-induced respiratory infections. J Manipulative Physiol Ther. 1999;22:530-533.

Griffin MD, Xing N, Kumar R. Vitamin D and its analogs as regulators of immune activation and antigen presentation. Annu Rev Nutr. 2003;23:117-145.

Griffiths RD, Jones C, Palmer TE. Six-month outcome of critically ill patients given glutamine-supplemented parenteral nutrition. Nutrition. 1997;13:295-302.

Hammer KA, Carson CF, Riley TV. Antimicrobial activity of essential oils and other plant extracts. J Appl Microbiol. 1999;86:985-990.

"Hand washing best defense against bird flu," Reuters via MSNBC.com, 21 November 2005.

Hassner A, Adelman DC. Biologic response modifiers in primary immunodeficiency disorders. Ann Intern Med. 1991;115:294-307.

Hathcock JN, Azzi A, Blumberg J, Bray T, Dickinson A, Frei B, Jialal I, Johnston CS, Kelly FJ, Kraemer K, Packer L, Parthasarathy S, Sies H, Traber MG. Vitamins E and C are safe across a broad range of intakes. Am J Clin Nutr. 2005;81:736-745. Review.

Hausen BM, Busker E, Carle R. The sensitizing capacity of composite plants. VII. Experimental studies with extracts and compounds of Chamomilla recutita (L.) Rauschert and Anthemis cotula L. Planta Med. 1984;50:229-234. German.

Helander IK, Alakomi HL, Latva-Kala K, Mattila-Sandholm T, Pol I, Smid EJ, von Wright A. Characterisation of the action of selected essential oil components on Gram-negative bacteria. J Agric Food Chem. 1998;46:3590-3595.

"HHS awards contracts totalling more than $1 billion to develop cell-based inflenza vaccine," U.S. Department of Health & Human Services, 4 May 2006. http://www.hhs.gov/news/press/2006pres/20060504.html. Accessed 4 May 2006.

"HHS Buys Additional Vaccine As Preparations For Potential Influenza Pandemic Continue," U.S. Department of Health & Human Services, 27 October 2005. http://www.hhs.gov/news/press/2005pres/20051027.html. Accessed 2 May 2006.

"HHS Buys Vaccine and Antivirals in Preparation for a Potential Influenza Pandemic," U.S. Department of Health & Human Services, 15 September 2005. http://www.hhs.gov/news/press/2005pres/20050915.html. Accessed 2 May 2006.

Hill LL, Woodruff LH, Foote JC, Barreto-Alcoba M. Esophageal injury by apple cider vinegar tablets and subsequent evaluation of products. J Am Diet Assoc. 2005;105:1141-1144.

Hollis BW. Circulating 25-hydroxyvitamin D levels indicative of vitamin D sufficiency: implications for establishing a new effective dietary intake recommendation for vitamin D. J Nutr. 2005;135:317-322.

"INFOSAN Information Note No. 7/2005 (Rev 1. 5 Dec) - Avian Influenza (Update of INFOSAN Information Note No. 2/04 - Avian Influenza, 17 Dec. 2004): Highly pathogenic H5N1 avian influenza outbreaks in poultry and in humans: Food safety implications," World Health Organization International Food Safety Authorities Network, 4 November 2005, http://www.who.int/entity/foodsafety/fs_management/No_07_AI_Nov05_en.pdf. Accessed 1 May 2006.

Janse A, and Gerba C. *The Germ Freak's Guide to Outwitting Colds and Flu.* Deerfield Beach, Fla: Health Communications Inc., 2005.

Josling P. Preventing the common cold with a garlic supplement: a double-blind, placebo-controlled survey. Adv Ther. 2001;18:189-193.

Kamath AB, Wang L, Das H, Li L, Reinhold VN, Bukowski JF. Antigens in tea-beverage prime human Vgamma 2Vdelta 2 T cells in vitro and in vivo for memory and nonmemory antibacterial cytokine responses. Proc Natl Acad Sci U S A. 2003;100:6009-6014.

Kelley KW, Brief S, Westly HJ, Novakofski J, Bechtel PJ, Simon J, Walker EB. GH3 pituitary adenoma cells can reverse thymic aging in rats. Proc Natl Acad Sci U S A. 1986;83:5663-5667.

Kelly GS. Larch arabinogalactan: clinical relevance of a novel immune-enhancing polysaccharide. Altern Med Rev. 1999;4:96-103.

Kim JM, Marshall MR, Wei CI. Antimicrobil activity of some essential oil components against five food-borne pathogens. J Agric Chem. 1995;43:2839-2845.

"Kimchi-spiced air conditions to fight bird flu," Reuters, 16 February 2006.

Kiskó G, Roller S. Carvacrol and p-cymene inactivate Escherichia coli O157:H7 in apple juice. BMC Microbiology. 2005;5:36.

Klatz R, Goldman R. *Infection Protection: How to Fight the Germs That Make You Sick.* New York: HarperCollins, 2002.

Klein SL, Wisniewski AB, Marson AL, Glass GE, Gearhart JP. Early exposure to genistein exerts long-lasting effects on the endocrine and immune systems in rats. Mol Med. 2002 Nov;8:742-749.

Knowles JR, Roller S, Murray DB, Naidu AS. Antimicrobial action of carvacrol at different stages of dual-species biofilm development by Staphylococcus aureus and Salmonella Typhimurium. Appl Env Microbiol. 2005;71:797-803.

Kodama N, Murata Y, Nanba H. Administration of a polysaccharide from Grifola frondosa stimulates immune function of normal mice. J Med Food. 2004;7:141-145.

Kriesel JD, Spruance J. Calcitriol (1,25-dihydroxy-vitamin D3) coadministered with influenza vaccine does not enhance humoral immunity in human volunteers. Vaccine. 1999;17:1883-1888.

Lardy H, Kneer N, Wei Y, Partridge B, Marwah P. Ergosteroids. II: Biologically active metabolites and synthetic derivatives of dehydroepiandrosterone. Steroids. 1998;63:158-165. Erratum in: Steroids 1999;64:497.

Laskova IL, Uteshev BS. [Immunomodulating action of heteropolysaccharides isolated from camomile flowers] Antibiot Khimioter. 1992;37:15-18. Russian.

LeBeau, C. J Immunity, vol 3 nr 4, Oct.-Dec. 2005.

Lee-Huang S, Zhang L, Huang PL, Chang YT, Huang PL. Anti-HIV activity of olive leaf extract (OLE) and modulation of host cell gene expression by HIV-1 infection and OLE treatment. Biochem Biophys Res Commun. 2003;307:1029-1037.

Legrand D, Elass E, Carpentier M, Mazurier J. Lactoferrin: a modulator of immune and inflammatory responses. Cell Mol Life Sci. 2005;62:2549-2559.

Li H, Xiong ST, Zhang SX, Liu SB, Luo Y. Immunological status of patients with obstructive jaundice and immunostimulatory effect of arginine. J Tongji Med Univ. 1993;13:111-115.

Lin R, White JH. The pleiotropic actions of vitamin D. Bioessays. 2004;26:21-28.

Lindenmuth GF, Lindenmuth EB. The efficacy of echinacea compound herbal tea preparation on the severity and duration of upper respiratory and flu symptoms: a randomized, double-blind placebo-controlled study. J Altern Complement Med. 2000;6:327-334.

Low TL, Thurman GB, Chincarini C, McClure JE, Marshall GD, Hu SK, Goldstein AL.Current status of thymosin research: evidence for the existence of a family of thymic factors that control T-cell maturation. Ann N Y Acad Sci. 1979;332:33-48.

Ma SC, He ZD, Deng XL, But PP, Ooi VE, Xu HX, Lee SH, Lee SF. In vitro evaluation of secoiridoid glucosides from the fruits of Ligustrum lucidum as antiviral agents. Chem Pharm Bull (Tokyo). 2001;49:1471-1473.

Maestroni GJ. Therapeutic potential of melatonin in immunodeficiency states, viral diseases, and cancer. Adv Exp Med Biol. 1999;467:217-226.

Maestroni GJ. The immunotherapeutic potential of melatonin. Expert Opin Investig Drugs. 2001;10:467-476.

Maestroni GJ. The photoperiod transducer melatonin and the immune-hematopoietic system. J Photochem Photobiol B. 1998;43:186-192.

Matsuda H, Murakami T, Ikebata A, Yamahara J, Yoshikawa M. Bioactive saponins and glycosides. XIV. Structure elucidation and immunological adjuvant activity of novel protojujubogenin type triterpene bisdesmosides, protojujubosides A, B, and B1, from the seeds of Zizyphus jujuba var. spinosa (Zizyphi Spinosi Semen). Chem Pharm Bull (Tokyo). 1999;47:1744-1748.

Melchart D, Linde K, Fischer P, Kaesmayr J. Echinacea for preventing and treating the common cold. [Review]. Cochrane Database Syst Rev. 2000;(2):CD000530.

Melhus H, Michaelsson K, Kindmark A, Bergstrom R, Holmberg L, Mallmin H, Wolk A, Ljunghall S. Excessive dietary intake of vitamin A is associated with reduced bone mineral density and increased risk for hip fracture. Ann Intern Med. 1998;129:770-778.

Messager S, Hammer KA, Carson CF, Riley TV. Effectiveness of hand-cleansing formulations containing tea tree oil assessed ex vivo on human skin and in vivo with volunteers using European standard EN 1499. J Hosp Infect. 2005;59:220-228.

Meydani SN, Meydani M, Blumberg JB, Leka LS, Siber G, Loszewski R, Thompson C, Pedrosa MC, Diamond RD, Stollar BD. Vitamin E supplementation and in vivo immune response in healthy elderly subjects. A randomized controlled trial. JAMA. 1997;277:1380-1386.

Michaelsson K, Lithell H, Vessby B, Melhus H. Serum retinol levels and the risk of fracture. N Engl J Med. 2003;348:287-294.

Miller ER 3rd, Pastor-Barriuso R, Dalal D, Riemersma RA, Appel LJ, Guallar E. Meta-analysis: high-dosage vitamin E supplementation may increase all-cause mortality. Ann Intern Med. 2005;142:37-46.

"Mixed success for Sanofi Pasteur's bird flu vaccine," SciDev.net, 11 May 2006.

Mori S, Ojima Y, Hirose T, Sasaki T, Hashimoto Y. The clinical effect of proteolytic enzyme containing bromelain and trypsin on urinary tract infection evaluated by double blind method. Acta Obstet Gynaecol Jpn. 1972;19:147-153.

Mossad SB. Effect of zincum gluconicum nasal gel on the duration and symptom severity of the common cold in otherwise healthy adults. QJM. 2003;96:35-43.

Nair N, Mahajan S, Chawda R, Kandaswami C, Shanahan TC, Schwartz SA. Grape seed extract activates Th1 cells in vitro. Clin Diagn Lab Immunol. 2002;9:470-476.

"National Strategy for Pandemic Influenza: Implementation Plan," U.S. White House. http://www.whitehouse.gov/homeland/pandemic-influenza-implementation.html. Accessed 3 May 2006.

"NIAID Initiates Trial of Experimental Avian Flu Vaccine," U.S. National Institute of Allergy and Infectious Diseases, March 23, 2005, http://www3.niaid.nih.gov/news/newsreleases/2005/avianfluvax.htm. Accessed 1 May 2006.

Nordvik I, Myhr KM, Nyland H, Bjerve KS. Effect of dietary advice and n-3 supplementation in newly diagnosed MS patients. Acta Neurol Scand. 2000;102:143-149.

Okamoto I, Taniguchi Y, Kunikata T, Kohno K, Iwaki K, Ikeda M, Kurimoto M. Major royal jelly protein 3 modulates immune responses in vitro and in vivo. Life Sci. 2003;73:2029-2045.

"OMT: Hands-On Care," American Osteopathic Association. http://www.osteopathic.org/index.cfm?PageID=ost_omt. Accessed 6 June 2006.

"Outbreak Notice: Human Infection with Avian Influenza A (H5N1) Virus," U.S. Centers for Disease Control & Prevention, issued 23 September 2005, http://www.cdc.gov/travel/other/avian_influenza_se_asia_2005.htm. Accessed 1 May 2006.

Park YC, Rimbach G, Saliou C, Valacchi G, Packer L. Activity of monomeric, dimeric, and trimeric flavonoids on NO production, TNF-alpha secretion, and NF-kappaB-dependent gene expression in RAW 264.7 macrophages. FEBS Lett. 2000;465:93-97.

Patterson M. "The coming influenza pandemic: lessons from the past for the future," Journal of the American Osteopathic Association, 105(11), November 2005, 498-500.

Pedrono F, Martin B, Leduc C, Le Lan J, Saiag B, Legrand P, Moulinoux JP, Legrand AB. Natural alkylglycerols restrain growth and metastasis of grafted tumors in mice. Nutr Cancer. 2004;48:64-69.

Pilotti V, Mastrorilli M, Pizza G, De Vinci C, Busutti L, Palareti A, Gozzetti G, Cavallari A. Transfer factor as an adjuvant to non-small cell lung cancer (NSCLC) therapy. Biotherapy. 1996;9:117-121.

Pizza G, De Vinci C, Cuzzocrea D, Menniti D, Aiello E, Maver P, Corrado G, Romagnoli P, Dragoni E, LoConte G, et al. A preliminary report on the use of transfer factor for treating stage D3 hormone-unresponsive metastatic prostate cancer. Biotherapy. 1996;9(1-3):123-32.

"Prevention of Avian Influenza," Hong Kong Government Information Center, 16 November 2005. http://www.info.gov.hk/info/flu/eng/faq.htm. Accessed 4 May 2006.

"Prevention of foodborne disease: Five keys to safer food," World Health Organization. http://www.who.int/foodsafety/consumer/5keys/en/index.html. Accessed 1 May 2006.

"Questions and Answers: H5N1 Avian Flu Vaccine Trials," U.S. National Institute of Allergy and Infectious Diseases, March 2006, http://www3.niaid.nih.gov/news/newsreleases/2005/H5N1QandA.htm. Accessed 1 May 2006.

Raso GM, Pacilio M, Di Carlo G, Esposito E, Pinto L, Meli R. In-vivo and in-vitro anti-inflammatory effect of Echinacea purpurea and Hypericum perforatum. J Pharm Pharmacol. 2002;54:1379-1383.

Raz R, Chazan B, Dan M. [Cranberry juice and urinary tract infection] Harefuah. 2004;143:891-894, 909.Hebrew.

Rehman J, Dillow JM, Carter SM, Chou J, Le B, Maisel AS. Increased production of antigen-specific immunoglobulins G and M following in vivo treatment with the medicinal plants Echinacea angustifolia and Hydrastis canadensis. Immunol Lett. 1999;68:391-395.

Reich S, Radenhausen M, Altmeyer P, Hoffmann K. [Extracorporeal photopheresis in progressive systemic sclerosis: discrimination of responders and non-responders]. J Dtsch Dermatol Ges. 2003;1:945-951. German.

Rogala E, Skopinska-Rozewska E, Sawicka T, Sommer E, Prosinska J, Drozd J. The influence of Eleuterococcus senticosus on cellular and humoral immunological response of mice. Pol J Vet Sci. 2003;6:37-39.

"Sauerkraut consumption may fight off breast cancer," NutraIngredients.com, 4 November 2005.

Scazzocchio F, Cometa MF, Tomassini L, Palmery M. Antibacterial activity of Hydrastis canadensis extract and its major isolated alkaloids. Planta Med. 2001;67:561-564.

Schauss AG, Vodjani A. Discovery of an edible fermentation product with unusual immune enhancing properties in humans. *FASEB J.* 2006; 20(4): A143).

Sheih YH, Chiang BL, Wang LH, Liao CK, Gill HS. Systemic immunity-enhancing effects in health subjects following dietary consumption of the lactic acid bacterium Lactobacillus rhamnosus HN001. J Am Coll Nutr. 2001;20:149-156.

Siddiqui YM, et al. Effect of essential oils on the enveloped viruses: antiviral activity of oregano oils on herpes simplex virus type I and Newcastle disease virus. Medical Sciences Research. 1996;24:185-186.

Sinclair S. Chinese herbs: a clinical review of Astragalus, Ligusticum, and Schizandrae. Altern Med Rev. 1998;3:338-344.

Sivropoulou A, Papanikolaou E, Nikolaou C, Kokkini S, Lanaras T, Arsenakis M. Antimicrobial and cytotoxic activities of oreganum essential oils. J Agric Food Chem. 1996;44:1202-1205.

Somasundar P, Riggs DR, Jackson BJ, Cunningham C, Vona-Davis L, McFadden DW. Inositol Hexaphosphate (IP6): A Novel Treatment for Pancreatic Cancer (1). J Surg Res. 2005;126:199-203.

"Statement of Jesse L. Goodman, M.D., M.P.H. Director, Center for Biologics Evaluation and Research before The Committee on Government Reform, U.S. Food and Drug Administration, February 10, 2005. http://www.fda.gov/ola/2005/influenza0210.html. Accessed 1 May 2006.

Stothers L. A randomized trial to evaluate effectiveness and cost effectiveness of naturopathic cranberry products as prophylaxis against urinary tract infection in women. Can J Urol. 2002;9:1558-1562.

Sutherland ER, Ellison MC, Kraft M, Martin RJ. Elevated serum melatonin is associated with the nocturnal worsening of asthma. J Allergy Clin Immunol. 2003;112:513-517.

Takagi Y, Choi IS, Yamashita T, Nakamura T, Suzuki I, Hasegawa T, Oshima M, Gu YH. Immune activation and radioprotection by propolis. Am J Chin Med. 2005;33:231-240.

"Today's bird flu vaccines will do," New Scientist News, 17 June 2006.

Tonks AJ, Cooper RA, Jones KP, Blair S, Parton J, Tonks A. Honey stimulates inflammatory cytokine production from monocytes. Cytokine. 2003;21:242-247.

Turner RB, Riker DK, Gangemi JD. Ineffectiveness of Echinacea for prevention of experimental rhinovirus colds. Antimicrob Agents Chemother. 2000;44:1708-1709.

"U.S. and World Population Clocks," U.S. Census Bureau, http://www.census.gov/main/www/popclock.html. Accessed 17 June 2006.

U.S. Centers for Disease Control & Prevention (CDC) Avian Flu website, http://www.cdc.gov/flu/avian/

U.S. Department of Health and Human Services (HHS) Pandemic Flu website, www.pandemicflu.gov

"USDA bans some French poultry due to highly pathogenic avian influenza," U.S. Department of Agriculture Animal and Plant Health Inspection Service, 27 February 2006, http://www.aphis.usda.gov/newsroom/content/2006/02/frenchai_vs.shtml. Accessed 1 May 2006.

Uteshev BS, Laskova IL, Afanas'ev VA. [The immunomodulating activity of the heteropolysaccharides from German chamomile (Matricaria chamomilla) during air and immersion cooling] Eksp Klin Farmakol. 1999;62:52-55. Russian.

"Vaccines for young may not work in the elderly," Medscape.com, May 12, 2006.

Valenti P, Antonini G. Lactoferrin: an important host defence against microbial and viral attack. Cell Mol Life Sci. 2005;62:2576-2587.

van Dissel JT, de Groot N, Hensgens CM, Numan S, Kuijper EJ, Veldkamp P, van 't Wout J. Bovine antibody-enriched whey to aid in the prevention of a relapse of Clostridium difficile-associated diarrhoea: preclinical and preliminary clinical data. J Med Microbiol. 2005;54:197-205.

van Hasselt P, Gashe BA, Ahmad J. Colloidal silver as an antimicrobial agent: fact or fiction? J Wound Care. 2004;13:154-155.

Vogel JU, Cinatl J, Dauletbaev N, Buxbaum S, Treusch G, Cinatl J Jr, Gerein V, Doerr HW. Effects of S-acetylglutathione in cell and animal model of herpes simplex virus type 1 infection. Med Microbiol Immunol (Berl). 2005;194:55-59.

Wagner H, Proksch A, Riess-Maurer I, Vollmar A, Odenthal S, Stuppner H, Jurcic K, Le Turdu M, Heur YH. [Immunostimulant action of polysaccharides (heteroglycans) from higher plants. Preliminary communication] Arzneimittelforschung. 1984;34:659-661. German.

Walsh DE, Griffith RS, Behforooz A. Subjective response to lysine in the therapy of herpes simplex. J Antimicrob Chemother. 1983;12:489-496.

Womble D, Helderman JH. The impact of acemannan on the generation and function of cytotoxic T-lymphocytes. Immunopharmacol Immunotoxicol. 1992;14:63-77.

Wu D, Meydani M, Leka LS, Nightingale Z, Handelman GJ, Blumberg JB, Meydani SN. Effect of dietary supplementation with black currant seed oil on the immune response of healthy elderly subjects. Am J Clin Nutr. 1999;70:536-543.

Wu JY, Gardner BH, Murphy CI, Seals JR, Kensil CR, Recchia J, Beltz GA, Newman GW, Newman MJ. Saponin adjuvant enhancement of antigen-specific immune responses to an experimental HIV-1 vaccine. J Immunol. 1992;148:1519-1525.

Yamamoto Y, Matsunaga K, Friedman H. Protective effects of green tea catechins on alveolar macrophages against bacterial infections. Biofactors. 2004;21:119-121.

Yellayi, S, A Naaz, MA Szewczykowski, T Sato, JA Woods, J Chang, M Segre, CD Allred, WG Helferich, PS Cooke. The phytoestrogen genistein induces thymic and immune changes: A human health concern? Proceedings of the National Academy of Sciences. 2002;99:7616-7621.

Young GA Jr, Underdahl NR, Carpenter LE. Vitamin D intake and susceptibility of mice to experimental swine influenza virus infection. Proc Soc Exp Biol Med. 1949;72:695-697.

Zakay-Rones Z, Thom E, Wollan T, Wadstein J. Randomized study of the efficacy and safety of oral elderberry extract in the treatment of influenza A and B virus infections. J Int Med Res. 2004;32:132-140.

Zhang CF, Yang P. Zinc-induced aggregation of Abeta (10-21) potentiates its action on voltage-gated potassium channel. Biochem Biophys Res Commun. 2006;345:43-49. Epub 2006 Apr 24.

Zuccotti GV, Salvini F, Riva E, Agostoni C. Oral lactoferrin in HIV-1 vertically infected children: an observational follow-up of plasma viral load and immune parameters. J Int Med Res. 2006;34:88-94.

CHAPTER 4

"Cholesterol-lowering drugs may be useful in an influenza pandemic," EurekAlert Press Release by Infectious Diseases Society of America, 13 June 2006.

Dean C. and Meininger E. "The history of influenza," totalhealth for Longevity, volume 7 number 5, February 2006, pgs 20-21.

"Drug shows promise against bird flu," Associated Press via baltimresun.com, 5 May 2006.

"Exploring flu drugs," U.S. National Institute of Allergy and Infectious Diseases, March 2006. http://www.niaid.nih.gov/factsheets/fludrugs.htm. Accessed 15 May 2006.

"Family quarantine is key to fighting bird flu," Kazinform, 27 April 2006, reporting on Nature Volume 440 Number 7088, pgs. 1089-1244.

"Flu drug Tamiflu fares well in testing," Associated Press via news.yahoo.com, 3 May 2006.

"GenoMed's Influenza ("Flu") & Avian Influenza ("Bird Flu") Trials," http://www.b2i.us/profiles/investor/fullpage.asp?f=1&BzID=571&to=cp&Nav=0&LangID=1&s=0 &ID=1159. Accessed 15 May 2006.

Greene J. *The Bird Flu Pandemic: Can it happen, will it happen?* New York: Thomas Dunne Books, 2006.

"Mass production of antiviral against bird flu," allheadlinenews.com, May 4, 2006.

Nature, volume 440 number 7088, pp. 1089-1244.

Sardi B. "What you should know about Tamiflu," 8 October 2005. http://www.knowledgeofhealth.com/report.asp?story=What%20You%20Should%20Know%20Abo ut%20Tamiflu&catagory=Infectious%20Disease,%20Vaccines,%20Flu,%20Drugs. Accessed 18 May 2006.

"Southeast Asia to have Tamiflu stockpile," AFX News Limited via Forbes.com, May 2, 2006.

"Statins may be helpful in bird flu pandemic," Science Daily, 13 June 2006. http://www.sciencedaily.com/upi/index.php?feed=Science&article=UPI-1-20060613-17195800-bc-us-birdflu-statins.xml. Accessed 14 June 2006.

U.S. Centers for Disease Control & Prevention (CDC) Avian Flu website, http://www.cdc.gov/flu/avian/.

U.S. Department of Health and Human Services (HHS) Pandemic Flu website, www.pandemicflu.gov.

CHAPTER 5

"Fact Sheet: Advancing the Nation's Preparedness for Pandemic Influenza," U.S. White House, 3 May 2006. http://www.whitehouse.gov/news/releases/2006/05/20060503-5.html. Accessed 3 May 2006.

"Family quarantine is key to fighting bird flu," Kazinform, 27 April 2006, reporting on Nature Volume 440 Number 7088, pgs. 1089-1244.

"HHS Pandemic Influenza Plan Fact Sheet," U.S. Department of Health & Human Services, 2 November 2005. http://www.hhs.gov/pandemicflu/plan/factsheet.html. Accessed 2 May 2006.

"National Strategy for Pandemic Influenza," U.S. White House, 1 November 2005. http://www.whitehouse.gov/homeland/pandemic-influenza.html. Accessed 2 May 2006.

"National Strategy for Pandemic Influenza: Implementation Plan," U.S. White House, 3 May 2006. http://www.whitehouse.gov/homeland/pandemic-influenza-implementation.html. Accessed 3 May 2006.

"New warnings on bird flu," The Week, 31 March 2006.

U.S. Centers for Disease Control & Prevention (CDC) Avian Flu website, http://www.cdc.gov/flu/avian/

U.S. Department of Health and Human Services (HHS) Pandemic Flu website, www.pandemicflu.gov

"U.S. plan for flu pandemic revealed," Washingtonpost.com, 16 April 2006.

"US outlines human bird flu plan," Reuters, 3 May 2006.

CHAPTER 6

"Exposure to Mumps During Air Travel --- United States," April 2006, MMWR, U.S. Centers for Disease Control & Prevention, April 11, 2006 / 55(Dispatch);1-2.

"Fact sheet: Basic information about SARS," U.S. Centers for Disease Control & Prevention, May 3, 2005.

"Global search for SARS vaccine gains momentum," World Health Organization, 5 November 2003.

"Inadequate plumbing systems likely contributed to SARS transmission," World Health Organization, 26 September 2003.

"Measles Alert; Updated June 7, 2006: Eleven Measles Cases Now Confirmed in Massachusetts," Massachusetts Department of Public Health (MDPH) Division of Epidemiology and Immunization, 7 June 2006.

"Mumps," U.S. Centers for Disease Control & Prevention, updated 18 May 2006.

"Mumps: Disease Q&A," U.S. Centers for Disease Control & Prevention, updated 18 May 2006.

"Report: Major cities not ready for catastrophe," Associated Press via NBC, 16 June 2006.

"UK Highest Level Of Measles In 20 Years," Allheadlinenews.com, 16 June 2006.

U.S. Centers for Disease Control & Prevention (CDC) Avian Flu website, http://www.cdc.gov/flu/avian/.

U.S. Department of Health and Human Services (HHS) Pandemic Flu website, www.pandemicflu.gov.

"Understanding Emerging and Re-Emerging Infectious Diseases," U.S. National Institute of Allergy and Infectious Diseases, October 1999.

"Virus turns killer as insect host fans out," New Scientist, 22 April 2006.

About the Authors

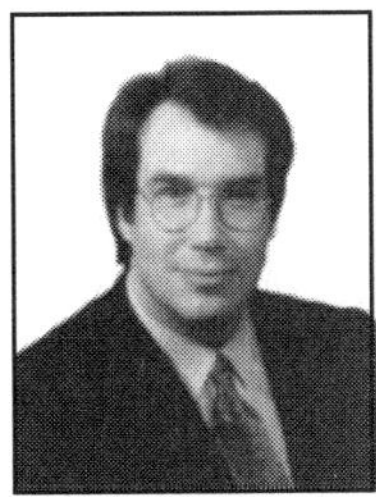

Ronald Klatz, M.D., D.O., who coined the term "anti-aging medicine," is recognized as a leading authority in the new clinical science of anti-aging medicine. Since 1981, Dr. Klatz has been integral in the pioneering exploration of new therapies for the treatment and prevention of age-related degenerative diseases. He is the physician founder and President of the American Academy of Anti-Aging Medicine Inc. ("A4M"), a non-profit medical organization dedicated to the advancement of technology to detect, prevent, and treat aging related disease and to promote research into methods to retard and optimize the human aging process. In his capacity as A4M President, Dr. Klatz oversees AMA/ACCME-approved continuing medical education programs for more than 30,000 physicians, health practitioners, and scientists from 85 countries worldwide.   He is instrumental in the continuing development of A4M's educational website, **www.worldhealth.net**, with an Internet audience exceeding 500,000 viewers, for which he serves as Senior Medical Editor.

Dr. Klatz co-founded the National Academy of Sports Medicine (NASM), which provides medical specialty training in musculoskeletal rehabilitation, conditioning, physical fitness, and exercise to 80,000 healthcare professionals internationally. He is a founder and key patent developer for Organ Recovery Systems, biomedical research company focusing on technologies for brain resuscitation, trauma and emergency medicine, organ transplant and blood preservation.

Dr. Klatz is the inventor, developer, or administrator of 100-plus scientific patents. In recognition of his pioneering medical breakthroughs, he was awarded the Gold Medal in Science for Brain Resuscitation Technology (1993) and the Grand Prize in Medicine for Brain Cooling Technology (1994). In addition, Dr. Klatz has been named as a Top 10 Medical Innovator in Biomedical Technology (1997) by the National Institute of Electromedical Information, and received the Ground Breaker Award in Health Care (1999) with Presidential Acknowledgment by William Jefferson Clinton from Transitional Services of New York.

The best selling author of 32 books with over 2 million copies in print, Dr. Klatz authored *Grow Young with HGH* (HarperCollins), *The New Anti-Aging Revolution, Stopping the Clock: Longevity for the New Millennium, Ten Weeks to a Younger You, New Anti-Aging Secrets for Maximum Lifespan, Brain Fitness* (Doubleday), *Hormones of Youth, Seven Anti-Aging Secrets, Advances in Anti-Aging, Stopping the Clock, Death in the Locker Room/Drugs & Sports, The E Factor, The Life Extension Weight Loss Program,* and *Deprenyl–The Anti Aging Drug* (partial list).

Dr. Klatz has served as a contributor, editor, reviewer and/or advisor to *Archives of Gerontology and Geriatrics, Journal of Gerontology, Osteopathic Annals Medical* Journal, *Patient Care Medical Journal, Total Health for Longevity,* and *50+ Plus* magazine. His columns on wellness and longevity have appeared in Pioneer Press (a division of Time-Life Inc), *Townsend Letter for Doctors and Patients, Spa Management Journal,* The Wellness Channel, *Fitness & Longevity Digest, Alternative Medicine Digest, Nutritional Science News, Healing Retreats & Spas, Skin Inc.,* and *Longevity SA* (for which he is served as Senior Medical Editor) (partial list).

Dr. Klatz has co-hosted the national Fox Network television series Anti-Aging Update and served as national advisor for Physician's Radio Network. He has appeared in interviews on CNN, USA Today TV, ABC News, NBC News, CBS News, Good Morning America, The Today Show, the Oprah Winfrey Show, Extra Daily TV News (partial list). Dr. Klatz has participated in articles appearing in the *New York Times, USA Today, Chicago Tribune, Newsweek, Harper's Bazaar, MacLean's* [Canada], *Forbes* Magazine, and *Investor's Business Daily* (partial list).

Dr. Klatz is highly regarded by scientific and academic colleagues for his continuing medical education lectures on the demographics of aging and the impact of biomedical technologies on longevity. His scientific articles have been published in *Resident and Staff Physician, British Journal of Sports Medicine, Medical Times/The Journal of Family Medicine, Osteopathic Annals,* and *American Medical Association News* (partial list).

Dr. Klatz is a graduate of Florida Technological University. He received the Doctor of Medicine (M.D.) Degree from the Central America Health Sciences University, School of Medicine, a government-sanctioned, Ministry of Health-approved, and World Health Organization-listed medical university. Dr. Klatz received his Doctor of Osteopathic Medicine and Surgery (D.O.) degree from the College of Osteopathic Medicine and Surgery (Des Moines, Iowa). Dr. Klatz is Board Certified in the specialties of Family Practice, Sports Medicine, and Anti-Aging Medicine.

Dr. Klatz has held several distinguished teaching or research positions, at Tufts University, the University of Oklahoma School of Osteopathic Medicine, Des Moines University School of Medicine, and the Chicago College of Osteopathic Medicine. Dr. Klatz is Professor, Department of Internal Medicine at the University of Central America Health Sciences. He has formerly served as Professor, Postgraduate Studies at Graduate School of Medicine at Swineburne University (Australia).

Publications
(continued)

2001
The Advanced Guide to Longevity Medicine
Editor

Anti-Aging Medical Therapeutics, volume IV
Editor

2000
New Anti-Aging Secrets for Maximum Lifespan
Author

Anti-Aging Medical Therapeutics, volume III
Editor

1999
Ten Weeks to a Younger You
Author

Brain Fitness (Doubleday)
Co-Author

1998
Hormones of Youth
Author

Grow Young with HGH (Harper Collins)
Author

Anti-Aging Therapeutics volume I
Editor

Anti-Aging Therapeutics, volume II
Editor

1996
Stopping the Clock – Therapies for Anti-Aging
Author

Seven Anti-Aging Secrets
Author

Advances in Anti-Aging Medicine - Textbook and Clinical Treatments
Author

1993
Deprenyl - The Anti-Aging Drug
Co-Author

1992
Drugs & Sports
Co-Author

The "E" Factor
Co-Author

About the Authors, *continued*

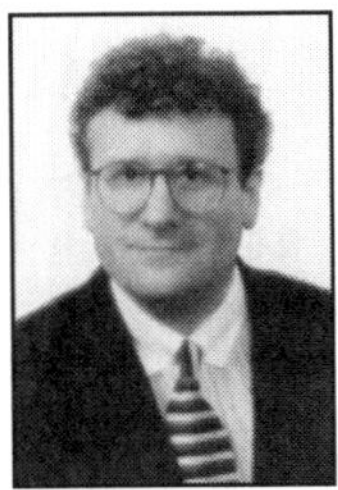

Robert M. Goldman M.D., Ph.D., D.O., FAASP has spearheaded the development of numerous international medical organizations and corporations. Dr. Goldman has served as a Senior Fellow at the Lincoln Filene Center, Tufts University, and as an Affiliate at the Philosophy of Education Research Center, Graduate School of Education, Harvard University. Dr. Goldman is Professor; Graduate School of Medicine, Swinburne University, Australia, and Clinical Consultant, Department of Obstetrics and Gynecology, Korea Medical University. He is also Professor, Department of Internal Medicine at the University of Central America Health Sciences, Department of Internal Medicine. Dr. Goldman is a Fellow of the American Academy of Sports Physicians and a Board Diplomat in Sports Medicine and Board Certified in Anti-Aging Medicine.

Dr. Goldman received his Bachelor of Science Degree (B.S.) from Brooklyn College in New York, then conducted three years of independent research in steroid biochemistry and attended the State University of New York. He received the Doctor of Medicine (M.D.) Degree from the Central America Health Sciences University, School of Medicine in Belize, a government-sanctioned, Ministry of Health-approved, and World Health Organization-listed medical university. He received his Doctor of Osteopathic Medicine and Surgery (D.O.) degree from Chicago College of Osteopathic Medicine at MidWestern University. His Ph.D. work was in the field of androgenic anabolic steroid biochemistry.

He co-founded and serves as Chairman of the Board of Life Science Holdings, a biomedical research company which has had over 150 medical patents under development in the areas of brain resuscitation, trauma and emergency medicine, organ transplant and blood preservation technologies. He has overseen cooperative research agreement development programs in conjunction with such prominent institutions as the American National Red Cross, the US National Aeronautics and Space Administration (NASA), the Department of Defense, and the FDA's Center for Devices & Radiological Health.

Dr. Goldman is the recipient of the 'Gold Medal for Science (1993), the Grand Prize for Medicine (1994), the Humanitarian Award (1995), and the Business Development Award (1996).

During the late 1990s, Dr. Goldman received honors from Minister of Sports and government Health officials of numerous nations. In 2001, Excellency Juan Antonio Samaranch awarded Dr. Goldman the International Olympic Committee Tribute Diploma for contributions to the development of sport & Olympism.

In addition, Dr. Goldman is a black belt in karate, Chinese weapons expert, and world champion athlete with over 20 world strength records, he has been listed in the Guinness Book of World Records. Some of his past performance records include 13,500 consecutive situps and 321 consecutive handstand pushups.

Dr. Goldman was an All-College athlete in four sports, a three time winner of the John F. Kennedy (JFK) Physical Fitness Award, was voted Athlete of the Year, was the recipient of the Champions Award, and was inducted into the World Hall of Fame of Physical Fitness. In 1995, Dr. Goldman was awarded the Healthy American Fitness Leader Award from the President's Council on Physical Fitness & Sports and U.S. Chamber of Commerce.

Dr. Goldman is Chairman of the International Medical Commission overseeing sports medicine committees in over 176 nations. He has served as a Special Advisor to the President's Council on Physical Fitness & Sports. He is founder and international President Emeritus of the National Academy of Sports Medicine and the cofounder and Chairman of the American Academy of Anti-Aging Medicine (A4M). Dr. Goldman visits an average of 20 countries annually to promote maximum human performance, brain research and sports medicine programs.

World Records Held by Dr. Goldman

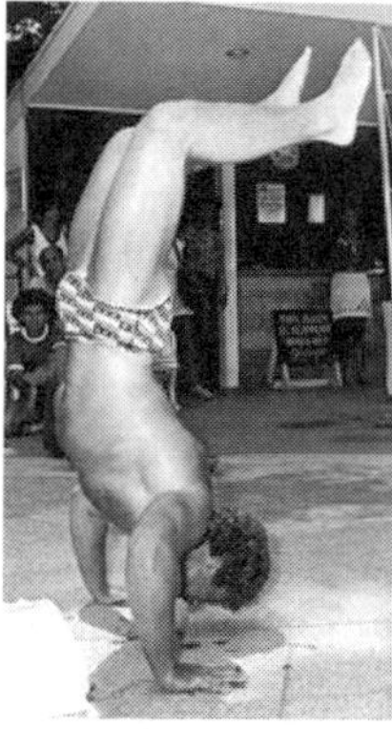

World Record
321 Consecutive
Handstand Pushups

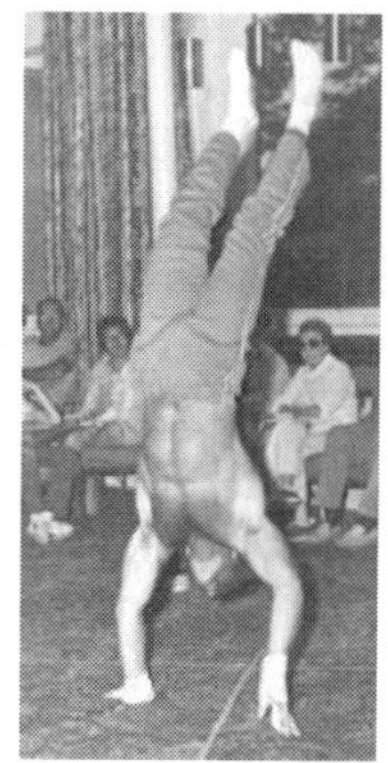

World Record
50-Yard Handstand
Sprint Trial

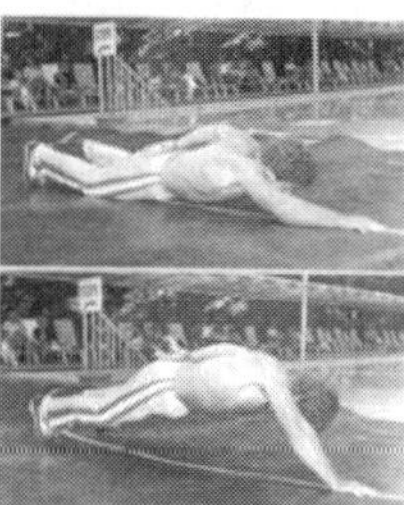

World Record
161 Consecutive
Overhead
Extension
One-Arm Pushups

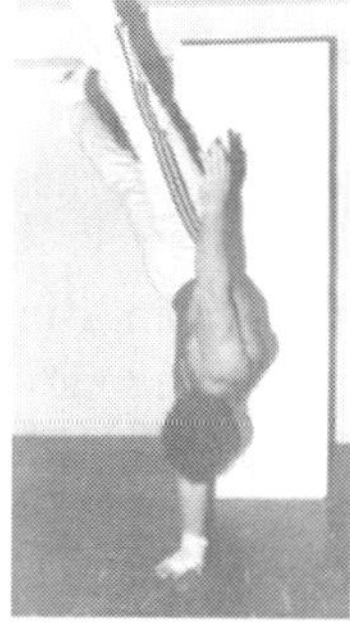

**One-Arm
Handstand
Pushup**

Dr. Goldman, President's Council on Physical Fitness & Sports

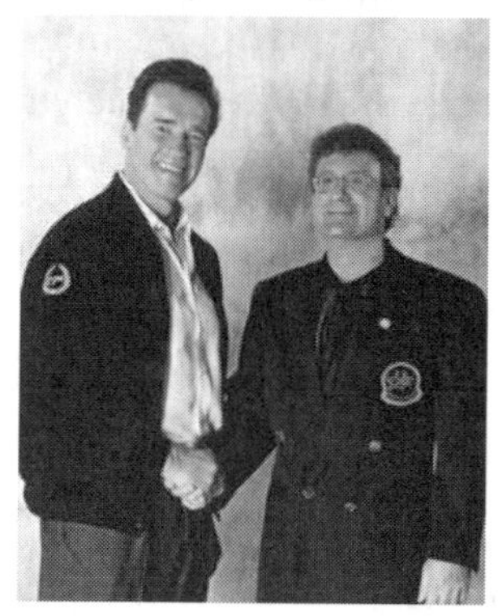

Dr. Goldman *(right)* served as Special Advisor to the President's Council on Physical Fitness & Sports under Governor Arnold Schwarzenegger's *(left)* Chairmanship of the Council.

Dr. Goldman, Recipient of the Gold Order of the International Federation of Body Builders (IFBB)

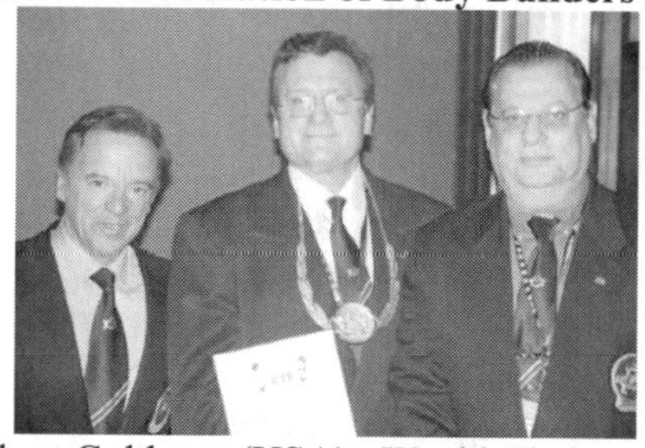

Dr. Robert Goldman (USA) , World Chairman IFBB Medical Commission, receives the IFBB's highest award - the IFBB Gold Order, at the World Championships in Shanghai, China, 2005
Shown here with Dr Rafael Santonja (Spain) past President of the Olympic Weight Lifting Federation of Spain, and Prof. Dr. Eduardo H. De Rose (Brazil), of the International Olympic Medical Commission.

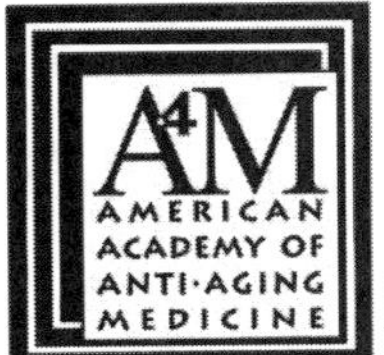

AMERICAN ACADEMY OF ANTI-AGING MEDICINE

1510 West Montana Street   Chicago, Illinois 60614 U.S.A.
Phone: (773) 528-4333   Fax: (773) 528-5390
e-mail: A4M@worldhealth.net

Internet: http://www.worldhealth.net

PRESIDENT
Ronald M. Klatz, M.D., D.O. - *USA*

CHAIRMAN OF THE BOARD
VICE PRESIDENT- NORTH AMERICA
Robert M. Goldman, M.D., Ph.D., D.O., FAASP - *USA*

VICE PRESIDENT - EUROPE
Rafael Santonja Gomez, Pharm.D.
Olympic Committee, Spain

VICE PRESIDENT - ASIA
Robert Tien, M.D., M.P.H. - *Taiwan*

CHAIRMAN - AMERICAN BOARD OF
ANTI-AGING MEDICINE (ABAAM)
Eduardo De Rose, M.D., Ph.D. - *Brazil*

EDUCATION SPECIAL ADVISOR -
AMERICAN BOARD OF ANTI-AGING
HEALTH PRACTITIONERS (ABAAHP)
Vernon A. Howard, Ph.D.
Harvard University (Ret.)

BOARD OF SCIENTIFIC ADVISORS
NORTH AMERICA
Denise Bruner, M.D. - *USA*
Past Pres., American Society of Bariatric Physicians
Louis Ignarro, Ph.D. - *USA*
1998 Nobel Laureate in Medicine
Shari Lieberman, Ph.D. - *USA*
University of Bridgeport (CT)
Stephen Sinatra, M.D. - *USA*
Manchester (CT) Medical Hospital
Robert Tan, M.D. - *USA*
University of Texas/Houston
Frederic Vagnini, M.D. - *USA*
Cornell University

ASIA-OCEANIA
Anon Chiangpradit, M.D. - *Thailand*
Dato Harnam, M.D., Ph.D. - *Malaysia*
Seung Ku, M.D., Ph.D. - *Korea*
Jan Matsuama, M.D. - *Japan*
Avni Sali, M.D., Ph.D. - *Australia*
S.K. Tan, M.D. - *Singapore*
Luis Vitetta, M.D., Ph.D. - *Australia*

EUROPE
Juan Marcos Becerro, M.D., Ph.D. - *Spain*
Vittorio Calabrese, M.D., Ph.D. - *Italy*
Thierry Hertoghe, M.D. - *Belgium*
Michael Klentze, M.D., Ph.D. - *Germany*

INFINITY AWARD RECIPIENTS
Roy Walford, M.D.
Caloric restriction mechanisms of aging
Nathan Pritikin, Ph.D.
Cholesterol and dietary risk factors for coronary artery disease
Linus Pauling, Ph.D.
Nobel Laureate
Vitamin C and megadose vitamins in health
Raymond Damadian, M.D.
Magnetic Resonance Image Scanner
Daniel Rudman, M.D.
Human Growth Hormone in aging
Karl Folkers, M.D.
Co-enzyme Q-10
Denham Harman, M.D., Ph.D.
Free radical theory of aging
Richard Cutler, Ph.D.
Role of antioxidants in aging
Peter Safar, M.D., Ph.D.
Cardiopulmonary Resuscitation
Senator John Glenn
Space and aging research
Judah Folkman, M.D.
Angiogenesis inhibitors for control of cancer
Representative Dan L. Burton
(US House of Representatives)
Advocacy of personal healthcare freedom
William Regelson, M.D.
Role of DHEA and melatonin in aging
Robert Atkins, M.D.
Role of obesity in aging
Ken Dychtwald, Ph.D.
Socio-economic implications of aging

A4M AustralAsia/Oceania
Jln. Moh Yamin I No. 9 Renon
Denpasar 80235
Bali - Indonesia
Phone: (62) 361 7494 180 or 190
Fax (62) 361 223 918
e-Fax (61) 733 196 527

HISTORY AND OVERVIEW

Anti-aging medicine is a medical specialty founded on the application of advanced scientific and medical technologies for the early detection, prevention, treatment, and reversal of age-related dysfunction, disorders, and diseases. It is a healthcare model promoting innovative science and research to prolong the healthy lifespan in humans. As such, anti-aging medicine is based on principles of sound and responsible medical care that are consistent with those applied in other preventive health specialties.

Mission:

The American Academy of Anti-Aging Medicine, Inc. ("A4M") is a non-profit medical organization dedicated to the advancement of technology to detect, prevent, and treat aging related disease and to promote research into methods to retard and optimize the human aging process. A4M is also dedicated to educating physicians, scientists, and members of the public on anti-aging issues. A4M believes that the disabilities associated with normal aging are caused by physiological dysfunction which in many cases are ameliorable to medical treatment, such that the human lifespan can be increased, and the quality of one's life improved as one grows chronologically older. A4M seeks to disseminate information concerning innovative science and research as well as treatment modalities designed to prolong the human lifespan. Anti-aging medicine is based on the scientific principles of responsible medical care consistent with those of other healthcare specialties. Although A4M seeks to disseminate information on any types of medical treatments, it does not promote or endorse any specific treatment nor does it sell or endorse any commercial product.

Membership

· Incorporated in 1993
· Membership of 18,500:
   · 85% physician members (M.D., D.O., and/or M.B.B.S.)
   · 12% scientist, researcher, and health practitioner members
   · 3% members of the working press and general public
· 85 nations represented

Objectives:

· Make available life-extending information about the multiple benefits of anti-aging therapeutics to practicing physicians.
· Assist in developing therapeutic protocols and innovative diagnostic tools to aid physicians in the implementation of effective longevity treatment.
· Act as an information center for valid and effective anti-aging medical protocols.
· Assist in obtaining and disseminating funding for scientifically sound and innovative research in anti-aging medicine.
· Assist in the funding and promotion of critical anti-aging, clinically based research.
· Government outreach, education, and advocacy for anti-aging medicine.

Core Activities:

· A4M trains over 30,000 physicians, health practitioners, and scientists annually at dozens of scientific conferences taking place in the United States and in venues worldwide.

Visit The World Health Network

www.worldhealth.net

The Official Website of the A4M

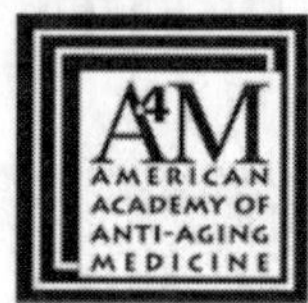

AMERICAN ACADEMY OF
ANTI-AGING MEDICINE (A4M)

New Membership / Renewal Application Form

Name : ....

Degrees : MD [] DO [] MBBS [] DC [] DDS [] ND [] PhD [] RPh [] RN [] NP [] PA [] Other : ....

Title : ....

Practice/Company : ....

Mailing Address : ....

City, State, Zip : ....

Country : ....

Phone : .... Fax : ....

Email : .... Website : ....

MEMBERSHIP CATEGORY

Membership Category	1 Year	2 Years	5 Years
[ ] Physician Membership (MD, DO, MBBS)	$150.00	$250.00	$500.00
[ ] Scientific/Healthcare (DC, DDS, ND, DPM, R.Ph, PhD, RN, NP, PA)	$95.00	$150.00	-
[ ] Preferred General Public	$89.95	-	-

I wish to be accepted as a member of the American Academy of Anti-Aging Medicine and agree to abide by its By Laws and Code of Ethics:

Signed : .... Date : ....

Please Select a Voluntary Contribution Level (optional) [ ] US$50 [ ] US$100 [ ] US$150 [ ] ....(Other)

Payment in the amount of US $ .... is enclosed (membership dues + contribution)

PAYMENT INFORMATION

Your membership will not be processed without full payment or if your credit card is declined.

[ ] Check # : .... payable to **A4M**, 1510 West Montana Street, Chicago, Illinois 60614, USA

[ ] Credit Card [ ] MC [ ] Visa [ ] AMEX Name on CC : ....

CC# : .... Security # : .... Expiry: ....

Signature : .... Date : ....

REMIT COMPLETED FORM TO:

____

Academy of Anti-Aging Medicine
1510 West Montana Street
Chicago, IL 60614 USA
Phone: 773-528-1000
Fax : 773-528-5390
Attn: **Membership Department**

Tracking Group# : _________________

- An Organizational Membership affords you extended benefits. Contact the A4M Membership Department for details.
- Allow 6-8 weeks for processing your new membership application and receipt of your Welcoming Kit and Member Certificate.
- Applicants wishing to return their A4M membership are required to comply to A4M.s
- Membership Return Policy. Instructions are available on the Membership. page at www.worldhealth.net and from the A4M
- Membership department.
- For inquiries, contact Customer Services at: **773-528-1000** or e-mail **membership@worldhealth.net**

You may also complete the On-Line Application Form
at The World Health Network

www.worldhealth.net
The Official Website of the A4M